2013
YEAR BOOK OF
UROLOGY®

The 2013 Year Book Series

Year Book of Critical Care Medicine®: Drs Dries, Zanotti-Cavazzoni, Latenser, Martinez, Rincon, and Zwank

Year Book of Emergency Medicine®: Drs Hamilton, Bruno, Handly, Minczak, Quintana, and Ramoska

Year Book of Endocrinology®: Drs Schott, Apovian, Clarke, Eugster, Meikle, Oetgen, Ovalle, Schteingart, and Toth

Year Book of Hand and Upper Limb Surgery®: Drs Yao, Adams, Isaacs, and Rizzo

Year Book of Medicine®: Drs Barker, Garrick, Gersh, Khardori, LeRoith, Panush, Talley, and Thigpen

Year Book of Neonatal and Perinatal Medicine®: Drs Fanaroff, Benitz, Donn, Neu, Papile, and Van Marter

Year Book of Neurology and Neurosurgery®: Drs Klimo, Minagar, Gandhi, Liu, Panagariya, Rezania, Riel-Romero, Riesenburger, Robottom, Schwendimann, Shafazand, and Yang

Year Book of Obstetrics, Gynecology, and Women's Health®: Drs Dungan and Shulman

Year Book of Oncology®: Drs Arceci, Bauer, Chiorean, Gordon, Lawton, Murphy, Thigpen, and Tsao

Year Book of Ophthalmology®: Drs Rapuano, Cohen, Flanders, Hammersmith, Milman, Myers, Nagra, Nelson, Penne, Pyfer, Sergott, Shields, Talekar, and Vander

Year Book of Orthopedics®: Drs Morrey, Huddleston, Rose, Swiontkowski, and Trigg

Year Book of Otolaryngology-Head and Neck Surgery®: Drs Sindwani, Balough, Franco, Gapany, and Mitchell

Year Book of Pathology and Laboratory Medicine®: Drs Raab and Bissell

Year Book of Pediatrics®: Dr Stockman

Year Book of Plastic and Aesthetic Surgery™: Drs Miller, Boehmler, Gosman, Gutowski, Ruberg, Salisbury, and Smith

Year Book of Psychiatry and Applied Mental Health®: Drs Talbott, Ballenger, Buckley, Frances, Krupnick, and Mack

Year Book of Pulmonary Disease®: Drs Barker, Jones, Maurer, Spradley, Tanoue, and Willsie

Year Book of Sports Medicine®: Drs Shephard, Cantu, Feldman, Galea, Jankowski, Janssen, Lebrun, and Nieman

Year Book of Surgery®: Drs Behrns, Daly, Fahey, Hines, Howe, Huber, Klodell, Mozingo, and Pruett

Year Book of Urology®: Drs Andriole and Coplen

Year Book of Vascular Surgery®: Drs Gillespie, Bush, Passman, Starnes, and Watkins

2013

The Year Book of UROLOGY®

Editors

Gerald L. Andriole, Jr, MD

Robert K. Royce Distinguished Professor, Chief of Urologic Surgery, Washington University School of Medicine, Barnes-Jewish Hospital, Siteman Cancer Center, St. Louis, Missouri

Douglas E. Coplen, MD

Associate Professor of Surgery (Urology), Washington University School of Medicine; Director of Pediatric Urology, St Louis Children's Hospital, St Louis, Missouri

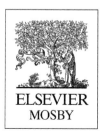

ELSEVIER
MOSBY

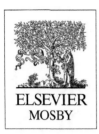

ELSEVIER
MOSBY

Vice President, Global Medical Reference: Mary Gatsch
Editor: Kerry Holland
Production Supervisor, Electronic Year Books: Donna M. Skelton
Electronic Article Manager: Mike Sheets
Illustrations and Permissions Coordinator: Dawn Vohsen

Printed and bound by CPI Group (UK) Ltd, Croydon, CR0 4YY
Transferred to digital print 2012

Editorial Office:
Elsevier
Suite 1800
1600 John F. Kennedy Blvd
Philadelphia, PA 19103-2899

International Standard Serial Number: 0084-4071
International Standard Book Number: 978-1-4557-7292-6

Contributors

J. Quentin Clemens, MD
Associate Professor of Urology; Director, Division of Neurourology and Pelvic Reconstructive Surgery, University of Michigan, Ann Arbor, Michigan

Adam S. Kibel, MD
Chief of Urology, Brigham and Women's Hospital; Professor of Urologic Surgery, Harvard Medical School, Boston, Massachusetts

Venkatesh Krishnamurthi, MD
Director, Kidney/Pancreas Transplant, Cleveland Clinic Foundation, Glickman Urological and Kidney Institute, Cleveland, Ohio

Eric S. Rovner, MD
Professor of Urology, Medical University of South Carolina; Attending Surgeon, Medical University Hospital, Charleston, South Carolina

Alan W. Shindel, MD
Assistant Professor, UC Davis School of Medicine, Sacramento, California

Jonathan M. Mobley, MD
Fellow, Endourology and Minimally Invasive Urology, Division of Urology, Washington University School of Medicine, St. Louis, Missouri

Youssef Tanagho, MD, MPH
Fellow, Minimally Invasive Urology, Washington University School of Medicine, St. Louis, Missouri

Contributors

Quentin Clemens, MD

Adam S. Kibel, MD

Venkatesh Krishnamurthi, MD

Moore, MD

Table of Contents

Journals Represented

Journals represented in this YEAR BOOK are listed below.

Acta Paediatrica
American Journal of Transplantation
British Journal of Cancer
British Journal of Psychiatry
British Journal of Urology International
Cancer
Cardiovascular and Interventional Radiological
Clinical Nuclear Medicine
European Journal of Obstetrics, Gynecology and Reproductive Biology
European Journal of Radiology
European Urology
Fertility and Sterility
Human Reproduction
International Brazilian Journal of Urology
International Journal of Radiation Oncology *Biology* Physics
Journal of Clinical Endocrinology & Metabolism
Journal of Clinical Oncology
Journal of Clinical Psychiatry
Journal of Endourology
Journal of Pediatric Surgery
Journal of Pediatric Urology
Journal of Sexual Medicine
Journal of the American Geriatrics Society
Journal of the American Medical Association Internal Medicine
Journal of the National Cancer Institute
Journal of Urology
Lancet
Mayo Clinic Proceedings
New England Journal of Medicine
Pediatrics
Proceedings of the National Academy of Sciences of the United States of America
Radiology
Urology

STANDARD ABBREVIATIONS

The following terms are abbreviated in this edition: acquired immunodeficiency syndrome (AIDS), cardiopulmonary resuscitation (CPR), central nervous system (CNS), cerebrospinal fluid (CSF), computed tomography (CT), deoxyribonucleic acid (DNA), electrocardiography (ECG), health maintenance organization (HMO), human immunodeficiency virus (HIV), intensive care unit (ICU), intramuscular (IM), intravenous (IV), magnetic resonance (MR) imaging (MRI), ribonucleic acid (RNA), ultrasound (US), and ultraviolet (UV).

NOTE

The YEAR BOOK OF UROLOGY is a literature survey service providing abstracts of articles published in the professional literature. Every effort is made to assure the accuracy of the information presented in these pages. Neither the editors nor the publisher of the YEAR BOOK OF UROLOGY can be responsible for errors in the original materials. The editors' comments are their own opinions. Mention of specific products within this publication does not constitute endorsement.

To facilitate the use of the YEAR BOOK OF UROLOGY as a reference tool, all illustrations and tables included in this publication are now identified as they appear in the original article. This change is meant to help the reader recognize that any illustration or table appearing in the YEAR BOOK OF UROLOGY may be only one of many in the original article. For this reason, figure and table numbers will often appear to be out of sequence within the YEAR BOOK OF UROLOGY.

1 Clinical Outcomes

Diagnosis, Evaluation and Follow-Up of Asymptomatic Microhematuria (AMH) in Adults: AUA Guideline
Davis R, Jones JS, Barocas DA, et al (American Urological Association Education and Res, Inc, Linthicum, MD)
J Urol 188:2473-2481, 2012

Purpose.—The purpose of this guideline is to provide a clinical framework for the diagnosis, evaluation and follow-up of asymptomatic microhematuria.

Materials and Methods.—A systematic literature review using the MEDLINE® database was conducted to identify peer reviewed publications relevant to the definition, diagnosis, evaluation and follow-up for AMH. The review yielded 191 evidence-based articles, and these publications were used to create the majority of the guideline statements. There was insufficient evidence-based data for certain concepts; therefore, clinical principles and consensus expert opinions were used for portions of the guideline statements.

Results.—Guideline statements are provided for diagnosis, evaluation and follow-up. The panel identified multiphasic computed tomography as the preferred imaging technique and developed guideline statements for persistent or recurrent AMH as well as follow-up.

Conclusions.—AMH is only diagnosed by microscopy; a dipstick reading suggestive of hematuria should not lead to imaging or further investigation without confirmation of three or greater red blood cells per high power field. The evaluation and follow-up algorithm and guidelines provide a systematic approach to the patient with AMH. All patients 35 years or older should undergo cystoscopy, and upper urinary tract imaging is indicated in all adults with AMH in the absence of known benign causation. The imaging modalities and physical evaluation techniques are evolving, and these guidelines will need to be updated as the effectiveness of these become available. Please visit the AUA website at http://www.auanet.org/content/media/asymptomatic_microhematuria_guideline.pdf to view this guideline in its entirety.

▶ Patients with hematuria make up a large component of urology and nephrology practices. The most common etiologies are infection, urinary calculi, and prostatic disease. Gross hematuria in adults is more likely indicative of pathology and nearly always requires evaluation (a less-extensive radiographic evaluation is indicated in children, and endoscopy is almost never performed). Often patients are referred for evaluation of a positive dipstick. However, if evaluation of the urinary sediment on more than one occasion shows no red cells, then the patient does not have microscopic hematuria and does not require further evaluation.

The real concern is that a small percentage of patients with asymptomatic microscopic hematuria will have a urinary tract malignancy. Risk factors, including age > 35 years, smoking history, occupational exposures, exposure to known carcinogens, coexisting irritative voiding symptoms, and foreign bodies, impact the extent of evaluation. The guidelines panel algorithm is detailed in the Fig of the original article. There is good evidence that the chance of developing a malignancy after an appropriate normal evaluation is very small. Most of the guideline recommendations are based on expert opinion and low-level clinical evidence. This does not limit the utility of the guidelines, as they are an excellent summary of the available literature and provide recommendations for appropriate clinical practice.

D. E. Coplen, MD

Long-Term Functional Outcomes after Treatment for Localized Prostate Cancer

Resnick MJ, Koyama T, Fan K-H, et al (Vanderbilt Univ, Nashville, TN; et al)
N Engl J Med 368:436-445, 2013

Background.—The purpose of this analysis was to compare long-term urinary, bowel, and sexual function after radical prostatectomy or external-beam radiation therapy.

Methods.—The Prostate Cancer Outcomes Study (PCOS) enrolled 3533 men in whom prostate cancer had been diagnosed in 1994 or 1995. The current cohort comprised 1655 men in whom localized prostate cancer had been diagnosed between the ages of 55 and 74 years and who had undergone either surgery (1164 men) or radiotherapy (491 men). Functional status was assessed at baseline and at 2, 5, and 15 years after diagnosis. We used multivariable propensity scoring to compare functional outcomes according to treatment.

Results.—Patients undergoing prostatectomy were more likely to have urinary incontinence than were those undergoing radiotherapy at 2 years (odds ratio, 6.22; 95% confidence interval [CI], 1.92 to 20.29) and 5 years (odds ratio, 5.10; 95% CI, 2.29 to 11.36). However, no significant between-group difference in the odds of urinary incontinence was noted at 15 years. Similarly, although patients undergoing prostatectomy were more likely to have erectile dysfunction at 2 years (odds ratio, 3.46; 95% CI, 1.93 to 6.17) and 5 years (odds ratio, 1.96; 95% CI, 1.05 to 3.63), no significant between-group difference was noted at 15 years. Patients undergoing prostatectomy were less likely to have bowel urgency at 2 years (odds ratio, 0.39; 95% CI, 0.22 to 0.68) and 5 years (odds ratio, 0.47; 95% CI, 0.26 to 0.84), again with no significant between-group difference in the odds of bowel urgency at 15 years.

Conclusions.—At 15 years, no significant relative differences in disease-specific functional outcomes were observed among men undergoing prostatectomy or radiotherapy. Nonetheless, men treated for localized prostate cancer commonly had declines in all functional domains during 15 years of follow-up. (Funded by the National Cancer Institute.)

▶ This was an elderly cohort of patients. At study inception, the median age was 64 in the prostatectomy group and 69 in the radiation group, which indicates that those median ages would now be 79 in the prostatectomy group and 84 in the radiation group. Fully 28% of the prostatectomy group and 50% of the radiation group died, leaving 842 prostatectomy subjects and 244 radiation subjects. Erectile dysfunction is now almost universal (85%–95% across all subjects). The raw numbers (Table in the original article) suggest that the findings from earlier analyses are still true (that urinary incontinence is still more common after prostatectomy than after radiation and that bowel dysfunction is still more common after radiation than after prostatectomy). However, after statistical adjustments, these values became virtually identical. The lack of a control group makes it difficult to know the degree to which aging contributed to the increase in symptoms over time in both treatment groups.

J. Quentin Clemens, MD

The 20-Year Public Health Impact and Direct Cost of Testosterone Deficiency in U.S. Men

Moskovic DJ, Araujo AB, Lipshultz LI, et al (Baylor College of Medicine, Houston, TX; New England Res Insts, Inc, Watertown, MA)
J Sex Med 2012 [Epub ahead of print]

Introduction.—Testosterone deficiency (TD) imposes a substantial public health burden in the U.S. We modeled the costs associated with TD-related sequelae including cardiovascular disease (CVD), diabetes mellitus (DM), and osteoporosis-related fractures (ORFs).

Aim.—To quantify the incremental cost burden imposed by TD's cardiometabolic sequelae.

Method.—Incidence, prevalence, and mortality of these conditions were collected for men ages 45–74 from six national databases and large cross-sectional studies. Relative risk (RR) rates were determined for these sequelae in patients with T < 300 ng/dL. The prevalence of TD was determined for this cohort of men.

Main Outcome Measures.—Adjusted incidence and prevalence were determined. Annual costs for the three TD-related sequelae were inflated at a real rate of 3% for 20 years.

Results.—Actual and adjusted (normalized for T deficiency) rates of CVD, DM, and ORFs in U.S. men aged 45–74 assuming a TD prevalence of 13.4% were calculated. We determined that, over a 20-year period, T deficiency is projected to be involved in the development of approximately

1.3 million new cases of CVD, 1.1 million new cases of DM, and over 600,000 ORFs. In year 1, the attributed cost burden of these diseases was approximately $8.4 billion. Over the entire 20-year period, T deficiency may be directly responsible for approximately $190–$525 billion in inflation-adjusted U.S. health care expenditures.

Conclusion.—TD may be a significant contributor to adverse public health. Further study is needed to definitively describe the whether TD is a modifiable risk factor for CVD, DM, and ORFs. This may represent an opportunity for nationwide public health initiatives aimed at preventive care.

▶ This interesting analysis estimates the health care costs of low testosterone, specifically costs associated with the higher rates of cardiovascular disease, diabetes, and bone fractures observed in men with testosterone levels below a threshold of 300 ng/dL.

This is a compelling article, but it's hard to know what to do with the results. Is testosterone deficiency in fact the driving factor in these health conditions? Will testosterone supplementation ameliorate these health conditions and their attendant costs? Is it legitimate to attribute the health care costs of diabetes mellitus (DM), fracture, or cardiovascular disease (CVD) to hypogonadism? Or is hypogonadism in some cases a side effect of other systemic illness? There is clear evidence that testosterone deficiency is associated with negative health outcomes, but it is far from complete. The authors mention this in their discussion section:

"Implicit in this analysis is the presumed causal role of T deficiency for CVD, DM, and osteoporosis. Emerging data will continue to clarify if T deficiency is in fact a preventable risk factor or rather a marker of disease. However, there is some preliminary evidence suggesting that lifestyle habits can influence T levels, thus suggesting the possibility of a folie a deux involving androgen status and metabolism."

Clearly, it is possible that 1 or more confounding variables (including lifestyle choices such as diet and exercise) may drive some of the association between hypogonadism and ill health.

This is a provocative analysis and timely given contemporary concerns about cost-effectiveness in health care. Further research will be required to determine the cost-effectiveness of testosterone treatment as a means to improve health care costs and outcomes in men. This will of course require more research to determine reasonable estimates of the benefits and risks (with respect to length and quality of life) that may be expected with testosterone supplementation in men. Will the final analysis demonstrate that screening and treating hypogonadism is effective at improving length/quality of life and cost-effective in improving length/quality of life? These are very important questions to ponder.

A. W. Shindel, MD

2 Imaging

Interactive magnetic resonance imaging for paediatric vesicoureteric reflux (VUR)
Arthurs OJ, Edwards AD, Joubert I, et al (Cambridge Univ Hosp NHS Foundation Trust, UK)
Eur J Radiol 82:e112-e119, 2013

Objectives.—The current gold standard for diagnosing vesicoureteric reflux in unsedated infants is the X-ray-based Micturating CystoUrethro-Gram (MCUG). The aim of this study was to assess the diagnostic performance of interactive MRI for voiding cysto-urethrography (iMRVC).

Methods.—25 infants underwent conventional MCUG followed by iMRVC. In iMRVC, patients were examined using a real-time MR technique, which allows interactive control of image contrast and imaging plane location, before, during and after micturition. Images were assessed for presence and grade of VUR. Parental feedback on both procedures was evaluated.

Results.—iMRVC gave a sensitivity of 100%, specificity of 90.5% (95% CI: 81.6–99.4%), PPV of 66.7% and NPV of 100% in this population. There was 88% concordance (44/50 renal units) according to the presence of VUR between the two methods, with iMRVC up-grading VUR in 6 units (12%). There was very good agreement regarding VUR grade: Kappa = 0.66 ± 0.11 (95% CI 0.43–0.88). 60% of parents preferred the MRI, but did not score the two tests differently.

Conclusion.—Interactive MRI allows dynamic imaging of the whole urinary tract without ionising radiation exposure. iMRVC gives comparable results to the MCUG, and is acceptable to parents.

▶ The authors demonstrate that magnetic resonance imaging (MRI) can be used to detect reflux and is comparable to the gold standard (voiding cystourethrogram [VCUG]). The figures show better spatial definition of reflux, but this is not necessarily information that is important in reflux management. Although the technique avoids the use of ionizing radiation, it still requires urethral catheterization. Parents, however, preferred the MRI because the infants did not need to be restrained during the MRI. In theory, this study could be combined with dynamic MR upper tract imaging. The technique is time intensive, and I would imagine very expensive when compared with the standard VCUG.

D. E. Coplen, MD

Development and Initial Validation of a Scoring System to Diagnose Testicular Torsion in Children

Barbosa JA, Tiseo BC, Barayan GA, et al (Boston Children's Hosp, MA; et al)
J Urol 189:1859-1864, 2013

Purpose.—Testicular torsion is a surgical emergency requiring prompt intervention. Although clinical diagnosis is recommended, scrotal ultrasound is frequently ordered, delaying treatment. We created a scoring system to diagnose testicular torsion, decreasing the indication for ultrasound.

Materials and Methods.—We prospectively evaluated 338 patients with acute scrotum, of whom 51 had testicular torsion. Physical examination was performed by a urologist, and all patients underwent scrotal ultrasound. Univariate analysis and logistic regression were performed, and a scoring system for risk stratification of torsion was created. Retrospective validation was performed with 2 independent data sets.

Results.—The scoring system consisted of testicular swelling (2 points), hard testicle (2), absent cremasteric reflex (1), nausea/vomiting (1) and high riding testis (1). Cutoffs for low and high risk were 2 and 5 points, respectively. Ultrasound would be indicated only for the intermediate risk group. In the prospective data set 69% of patients had low, 19% intermediate and 11.5% high risk. Negative and positive predictive values were 100% for cutoffs of 2 and 5, respectively (specificity 81%, sensitivity 76%). Retrospective validation in 1 data set showed 66% of patients at low, 16% intermediate and 17% high risk. Negative and positive predictive values for cutoffs of 2 and 5 were 100% (specificity 97%, sensitivity 54%). The second retrospective data set included only torsion cases, none of which was misdiagnosed by the scoring system.

Conclusions.—This scoring system can potentially diagnose or rule out testicular torsion in 80% of cases, with high positive and negative predictive values for selected cutoffs. Ultrasound orders would be decreased to 20% of acute scrotum cases. Prospective validation of this scoring system is necessary.

▶ The TWIST (testicular workup for ischemia and suspected torsion) study develops a scoring system to help predict the need for imaging or surgical exploration in boys with testicular pain. Surprisingly, the average duration of symptoms before evaluation at Boston Children's Hospital was 72 hours. This alone makes it less likely that the boys were being evaluated for acute testicular torsion. Indeed, two-thirds of the patients were deemed low risk based on the criteria in the scoring system. The results may differ if a subset of patients presenting acutely was evaluated.

I find that the real issue is that primary care and emergency room (ER) physicians have different physical examination skills and a different threshold for ordering tests and consulting urologists. From my standpoint, this scoring system would be more useful if it was created and validated in a primary or ER setting. This would further decrease the overutilization of scrotal imaging in boys with scrotal pain. Urologists need to be involved in indeterminate and surgical cases. Ultrasound scan can be selectively utilized in cases in which the history and urologic examination are discordant.

D. E. Coplen, MD

3 Quality Improvement

Unintended Consequences of Eliminating Medicare Payments for Consultations

Song Z, Ayanian JZ, Wallace J, et al (Harvard Med School, Boston, MA; Harvard Univ, Cambridge, MA)
JAMA Intern Med 173:15-21, 2013

Background.—Prior to 2010, Medicare payments for consultations (commonly billed by specialists) were substantially higher than for office visits of similar complexity (commonly billed by primary care physicians). In January 2010, Medicare eliminated consultation payments from the Part B Physician Fee Schedule and increased fees for office visits. This change was intended to be budget neutral and to decrease payments to specialists while increasing payments to primary care physicians. We assessed the impact of this policy on spending, volume, and complexity for outpatient office encounters in 2010.

Methods.—We examined outpatient claims from 2007 through 2010 for 2 247 810 Medicare beneficiaries with Medicare Supplemental (Medigap) coverage through large employers in the Thomson Reuters MarketScan Database. We used segmented regression analysis to study changes in spending, volume, and complexity of office encounters adjusted for age, sex, health status, secular trends, seasonality, and hospital referral region.

Results.—"New" office visits largely replaced consultations in 2010. An average of $10.20 more was spent per beneficiary per quarter on physician encounters after the policy (6.5% increase). The total volume of physician encounters did not change significantly. The increase in spending was largely explained by higher office-visit fees from the policy and a shift toward higher-complexity visits to both specialists and primary care physicians.

Conclusions.—The elimination of consultations led to a net increase in spending on visits to both primary care physicians and specialists. Higher prices, partially owing to the subjectivity of codes in the physician fee schedule, explained the spending increase, rather than higher volumes.

▶ In January 2010, the Centers for Medicare and Medicaid Services eliminated payments for evaluation and management (E&M) codes for office consultations. At the same time, fees for regular office visits (billed more frequently by primary care physicians) were increased. The goal of these changes was to increase reimbursement for primary care providers, at the expense of specialists. The underlying rationale is that such changes would help drive more medical student interest in primary care and ultimately would help reduce the primary care shortage. These authors found that these 2010 changes caused an increase in overall Medicare spending, whereas initial projections had suggested that these changes would be budget neutral and would not increase spending. The increase in overall spending was driven by up-coding of office visits after 2010 by both primary care providers and specialists.

One very important factor that was not discussed by the authors is the adoption of electronic medical record (EMR) systems, which has been increasingly occurring because of the implementation of various government incentives. The adoption of EMRs may lead to up-coding for E&M services because accurate documentation is facilitated by the EMR systems. Therefore, it is possible that implementation of EMRs was at least partially responsible for the increase in overall Medicare spending, as opposed to elimination of the consultation visit. Regarding the up-coding controversy, it is worthwhile to note that the most aggressive billing practices have been observed in physicians practicing family medicine, internal medicine, and emergency medicine.[1]

J. Quentin Clemens, MD

Reference

1. Levinson, D. Coding Trends of Medicare Evaluation and Management Services. May 2012. https://oig.hhs.gov/oei/reports/oei-04-10-00180.pdf. Accessed May 28, 2013.

4 Clinical Research

Aspiration and Sclerotherapy: A Nonsurgical Treatment Option for Hydroceles
Francis JJ, Levine LA (Rush Univ Med Ctr, Chicago, IL)
J Urol 189:1725-1729, 2013

Purpose.—We demonstrated that hydrocele aspiration and sclerotherapy with doxycycline is an effective and safe nonsurgical treatment option for hydrocele correction.

Materials and Methods.— The medical records of patients who underwent hydrocele aspiration and sclerotherapy were analyzed in a retrospective cohort study for success rates as well as improvement in scrotal size and discomfort after a single hydrocele aspiration and sclerotherapy treatment. Patients who reported decreased scrotal size, improved physical symptoms and satisfaction with the procedure were considered as having success with hydrocele aspiration and sclerotherapy.

Results.—A total of 29 patients (mean age 52.8 years) presenting with 32 nonseptated hydroceles underwent hydrocele aspiration and sclerotherapy with doxycycline between 2005 and 2012. Of the hydroceles 27 (84%) were successfully treated with a single aspiration and sclerotherapy procedure. Overall mean followup was 20.8 months. Three patients reported moderate pain which resolved in 2 to 3 days. Of those patients in whom hydrocele aspiration and sclerotherapy failed, 1 had hydrocele successfully resolved with a second aspiration and sclerotherapy treatment, 3 did not have success with a second procedure and underwent hydrocelectomy, and 1 wanted immediate surgical correction.

Conclusions.—Hydrocele aspiration and sclerotherapy was successful in correcting 84% of simple nonseptated hydroceles with a single treatment. This result is an increase from previously reported success rates involving a single hydrocele aspiration and sclerotherapy procedure with tetracycline (75%). The success rate of a single hydrocele aspiration and sclerotherapy procedure is similar to the reported success rates involving hydrocelectomy while avoiding the hospital expense and many other complications. We conclude that the hydrocele aspiration and sclerotherapy procedure is a reasonable, nonsurgical and underused treatment option for nonseptated simple hydroceles.

▶ The authors aspirated (using a 16-gauge angiocath) and sclerosed hydroceles using doxycycline diluted in 10 mL of 0.5% bupivacaine without epinephrine. The scrotum was massaged for a minute after instillation to diffuse the doxycycline.

11

In most men the scrotum returned to normal size within 4 to 6 months. Success was excellent with nearly 2-year follow-up. All men were given a narcotic prescription after the procedure, but there is no quantification of the magnitude of pain, length of discomfort, and narcotic utilization.

The cost savings when comparing aspiration with surgical hydrocelectomy are huge. The estimated charges for aspiration are $459 and operative management are $12 300 (Table 2 in the original article). This becomes increasingly important as costs and patient outcomes impact physician reimbursement. This approach is promising. A controlled trial would elucidate the utility of hydrocele aspiration.

D. E. Coplen, MD

5 Endourology and Stone Disease

Endourology

Prospective Evaluation and Classification of Ureteral Wall Injuries Resulting from Insertion of a Ureteral Access Sheath During Retrograde Intrarenal Surgery

Traxer O, Thomas A (Univ Pierre and Marie Curie, Paris, France; Univ Hosp of Liége, Belgium)

J Urol 189:580-584, 2013

Purpose.—The safety of using a ureteral access sheath during retrograde intrarenal surgery remains controversial. Using a novel classification, we prospectively evaluated the incidence and severity of ureteral access sheath driven ureteral wall injury after flexible ureteroscopy for retrograde intrarenal surgery.

Materials and Methods.—Data on a total of 359 consecutive patients who underwent retrograde intrarenal surgery for kidney stone were prospectively collected at 2 academic centers. We propose what is to our knowledge a novel endoscopic classification of iatrogenic ureteral wall injury. Ureteral injuries after retrograde intrarenal surgery were assessed visually with a digital flexible ureterorenoscope. The primary outcome measure was the incidence and nature of ureteral injuries. We sought factors predisposing to such injuries.

Results.—Ureteral wall injury was found in 167 patients (46.5%). Severe injury involving the smooth muscle layers was observed in 48 patients (13.3%). Males vs females ($p = 0.024$) and older vs younger patients ($p = 0.018$) were at higher risk for severe ureteral access sheath related ureteral injury. The most significant predictor of severe injury was absent ureteral Double-J® stenting before retrograde intrarenal surgery ($p < 0.0001$). Pre-stenting vs no pre-stenting decreased the risk of severe injury by sevenfold. Body mass index, a history of diabetes mellitus, vascular disease or abdominopelvic radiation therapy and operative time were not associated with severe ureteral injury.

Conclusions.—Ureteral access sheath use for retrograde intrarenal surgery should involve systematic visual assessment of the entire ureter to recognize severe ureteral injury. The incidence of severe ureteral injury is largely decreased by preoperative Double-J stenting.

▶ Based on the data in this article, a ureteral access sheath (UAS) generates significant shear forces in the ureter. The appendix delineates a classification of ureteral injury that is based on mucosal, muscular, or full-thickness ureteral injury identified after placement of a ureteral access sheath. The figure in the article gives clear endoscopic images of 3 ureteral injury grades. Grade 2 (mucosal and smooth muscle injury) was identified in 10% of patients. Grade 3 (full-thickness injury with visualization of periureteral fat) occurred in 3%. There were no ureteral avulsions. All patients underwent stent placement after UAS. There is no long-term follow-up to assess if these ureteral injuries led to ureteral strictures. Placement of a stent to allow passive dilation before placement of a UAS decreases the incidence of severe (grade 2 and 3) injury, but placement requires a second anesthetic, and stents alone can cause significant patient morbidity. Because the UAS is not benign, utilization should be selective and done with caution.

D. E. Coplen, MD

Contemporary Management of Ureteral Stones

Bader MJ, Eisner B, Porpiglia F, et al (Ludwig-Maximilians-Univ, Munich, Germany; Massachusetts General Hosp, Boston; Universitá degli Studi di Torino, Italy; et al)
Eur Urol 61:764-772, 2012

Context.—Ureteral calculi represent a common condition that urologists encounter in everyday practice. Several treatment options are available for calculi that do not pass spontaneously or are unlikely to do so.

Objective.—In this nonsystematic review, we summarize the existing data on contemporary management of ureteral stones focusing on medical expulsive therapy (MET) and different treatment modalities.

Evidence Acquisition.—A PubMed search was performed. We reviewed the recent literature on the management of ureteral calculi. Articles were considered between 1997 and 2011. Older studies were included selectively if historically relevant.

Evidence Synthesis.—For stones that do not pass spontaneously or with MET, shock wave lithotripsy (SWL) and ureteroscopy (URS) are the most common and efficient treatment modalities. Both techniques have obvious advantages and disadvantages as well as different patterns of complications. For select cases or patients, other modalities may be useful.

Conclusions.—Ureteral stones of up to 10 mm and eligible for observation may be offered MET. For most ureteral calculi that require treatment, advances in SWL and URS allow urologists to take a minimally invasive approach. Other more invasive treatments are reserved for select "nonstandard" cases.

▶ This article provides an up-to-date review of the current management of ureteral stones. A nonsystematic review of the literature was performed using PubMed and the Cochrane Library. The majority of the articles were chosen from 1997 to 2011. Overall summaries of the sections are as follows.

Medical expulsive therapy (MET) is an option for ureteral stones less than 10 mm in size. The use of calcium channel blockers or α-adrenergic antagonist is associated with a greater likelihood of stone passage, shorter time to stone passage, and decreased pain scores. At this time, no superiority between calcium channel blockers and α-adrenergic antagonist is known.

Acceptable first-line therapies for ureteral stones include both extracorporeal shock wave lithotripsy (SWL) and ureteroscopy (URS). For proximal stones less than 10 mm, SWL was superior to URS (90% vs 80%). Prestenting is not required for SWL since outcomes are not improved. For proximal stones greater than 10 mm, SWL was inferior to URS (68% to 79%). In the midureter, URS is likely to have a higher success rate. The American Urological Association/ European Association of Urology Nephrolithiasis Guideline Panel states "Stenting following uncomplicated ureteroscopy is optional." Finally, ureteral stenting has shown benefit following the use of a ureteral access sheath.

This article also reviews populations with unique needs, such as children, pregnant women, and patients with a coagulopathy or on anticoagulation medications. For children, both SWL and URS are effective treatment options with proper equipment and clinical training. Pregnant women can be managed conservatively or with temporizing measures such as stents and nephrostomy drainage. Stents and nephrostomy tubes should be changed to prevent encrustation. Ureteroscopy is another safe option for evaluation and treatment of stones in pregnant women. Patients with coagulopathies or on anticoagulation medication should undergo ureteroscopy with laser lithotripsy if treatment is required. Percutaneous antegrade ureteroscopy can be first-line treatment in a few situations: additional large renal stone burden, a large ureteropelvic stone or upper ureteral stone, patients with urinary diversion, and men with large prostates that fail SWL. Finally, open and laparoscopic techniques are only considered in "extreme situations or in cases of simultaneous open surgery for another purpose."

J. M. Mobley, MD

A single dose of a non-steroidal anti-inflammatory drug (NSAID) prevents severe pain after ureteric stent removal: A prospective, randomised, double-blind, placebo-controlled trial
Tadros NN, Bland L, Legg E, et al (Oregon Health & Science Univ, Portland; et al)
BJU Int 111:101-105, 2013

Objectives.—• To determine the incidence of severe pain after ureteric stent removal.

• To evaluate the efficacy of a single dose of a non-steroidal anti-inflammatory drug (NSAID) in preventing this complication.

Patients and Methods.—• A prospective, randomised, double-blind, placebo-controlled trial was performed at our institution.

• Adults with an indwelling ureteric stent after ureteroscopy were randomised to receive either a single dose of placebo or an NSAID (rofecoxib 50 mg) before ureteric stent removal.

• Pain was measured using a visual analogue scale (VAS) just before and 24 h after stent removal

• Pain medication use after ureteric stent removal was measured using morphine equivalents.

Results.—• In all, 22 patients were enrolled and randomised into the study before ending the study after interim analysis showed significant decrease in pain level in the NSAID group.

• The most common indication for ureteroscopy was urolithiasis (14 patients).

• The proportion of patients with severe pain (VAS score of ≥ 7) during the 24 h after ureteric stent removal was six of 11 (55%) in the placebo group and it was zero of 10 in the NSAID group ($P < 0.01$).

• There were no complications related to the use of rofecoxib.

Conclusions.—• We found a 55% incidence of severe pain after ureteric stent removal.

• A single dose of a NSAID before stent removal prevents severe pain after ureteric stent removal.

▶ Even though stents were left in situ for more than 2 weeks after therapeutic ureteroscopy, most patients in the placebo group had severe pain after stent removal. Despite the small sample size, analgesic use was statistically higher in the subset with severe pain, although there was no difference in pain medication when comparing all patients in the 2 groups. Inflammation and ureteral orifice edema are the presumed etiology of the discomfort. It is unclear why a single dose of a nonsteroidal anti-inflammatory drug (NSAID) immediately decreases pain, as resolution of the edema would take hours or days. The mechanism must be related to blockage of prostaglandin synthesis and reduction in renal pelvic and ureteral pressure (by reducing renal blood flow). A single dose of an NSAID administered before stent removal is safe and may decrease acute pain after stent removal.

D. E. Coplen, MD

Association Between Obstructive Sleep Apnea and Urinary Calculi: A Population-based Case-control Study

Kang J-H, Keller JJ, Chen Y-K, et al (Taipei Med Univ Hosp, Taiwan; Taipei Med Univ, Taiwan; et al)
Urology 79:340-345, 2012

Objective.—To hypothesize an association between obstructive sleep apnea (OSA) and urinary calculi (UC) and assess the presence of such an association using a national population-based dataset. Elevated systemic proinflammatory pathways found in OSA patients may be linked to increased cardiovascular risk. Similar pathways have been identified in patients with UC.

Materials and Methods.—We identified 53,791 patients who had received a new diagnosis of UC between 2003 and 2008 from a dataset based on Taiwan's National Health Insurance program. We randomly selected 161,373 controls and then identified subjects with prior OSA in both groups. Odds ratios (ORs) for prior OSA in UC patients compared with controls were estimated in conditional logistic regression analyses by sex and by age group.

Results.—Prevalences of prior OSA were 1.2% in all subjects, 1.5% in patients with UC, and 1.1% in controls. After adjusting for patients' monthly income, geographic location, urbanization level, hypertension, diabetes, coronary heart disease and hyperlipidemia, and obesity, the OR for prior OSA in UC patients was 1.38 (95% CI 1.30-1.49) compared with controls. Prior OSA was associated with UC both in both males (OR 1.30, 95% CI 1.18-1.41) and females (OR 1.45, 95% CI 1.22-1.67). Notably, the adjusted OR was most pronounced in the youngest age group, <35 years (OR 2.57, 95% CI 1.97-3.34).

Conclusions.—We conclude that patients with UC had a higher prevalence of prior OSA. The OR for prior OSA was most pronounced in the youngest age group.

▶ These authors are the first to suggest an association of obstructive sleep apnea (OSA) with urinary calculi (UC). A case-control study was performed using insurance data from the Taiwan Longitudinal Health Insurance Database (LHID2000) The study gathered information from 53791 patients with newly diagnosed UC and 161 373 controls. The rates of OSA were compared for the 2 groups. Regression modeling was used to adjust for sex, age, monthly income, geographic location, urbanization level, hypertension, diabetes, coronary heart disease, hyperlipidemia, and obesity. After the above adjustments, the UC group was found to have a higher risk of OSA compared to the control (odds ratio [OR] 1.38; 95% confidence interval [CI], 1.3–1.49; $P < .001$). These findings were more pronounced in the female population (OR 1.45; 95% CI, 1.22–1.67; $P < .001$) and in patients younger than 35 years of age (OR 2.57; 95% CI, 1.97–3.34; $P < .01$).

The etiology for this trend is currently unknown. These authors propose that obesity and the presence of metabolic syndrome could contribute to this association. In this case, when using binary variables for obesity, diabetes, hypertension, and hyperlipidemia, OSA was still more prevalent in the UC group compared with the controls. Hopefully, future investigations will prove or disprove this association in populations outside of Taiwan and also exclude further secondary variables.

J. M. Mobley, MD

Impact of Radiological Technologists on the Outcome of Shock Wave Lithotripsy

Elkoushy MA, Morehouse DD, Anidjar M, et al (McGill Univ, Montreal, Quebec, Canada)
Urology 79:777-780, 2012

Objective.—To evaluate the correlation of radiological technologists (RTs) and the outcome of shock wave lithotripsy (SWL) in terms of fluoroscopy time, fragmentation rate, and stone-free rate.

Material and Methods.—A retrospective review of a prospectively collected database of 601 SWL treatments between June 2009 and March 2010 was performed. Patients with radiolucent stones were excluded. SWL was done by 6 RTs with different levels of experience. Follow up was available for 534 treatments. Multivariate analysis was performed.

Results.—RTs (A-F) performed 144, 109, 118, 58, 57, and 48 SWL sessions, respectively. There was no statistical difference among RTs in terms of mean stone size or stone location. Compared with other RTs, RT A had a significantly lower mean fluoroscopy time of 129 seconds (95% CI 120.8-137.3) (P <.001), higher stone-free rate (75.7%; P =.035), and stone fragmentation rate after a single SWL session (82.6%; P =.004). After correcting for stone size and location, fluoroscopy time (P <.001), fragmentation rate (P =.002), and stone-free rate (P =.04) maintained their significance. When comparing the top 3 RTs performing >100 SWL sessions, RTs B and C had significantly higher fluoroscopy time compared with RT A (OR [95% CI] 1.84 [1.38-2.45]; P <.001 and 2.67 [2.00-3.57]; P <.001), respectively. After correcting for stone size and location, RT B had significantly lower fragmentation rate when compared with RT A (OR [95% CI] 0.21 [0.05-0.86], P =.03]. However, there were no significant differences among the top 3 RTs in terms of stone-free rates.

Conclusion.—RTs significantly differ in fluoroscopy usage in addition to stone fragmentation and stone-free rates (Table 2).

▶ Prior investigations show that final outcomes for shock wave lithotripsy (SWL) vary with the urologist's experience. This study instead focused on the radiologic technologist's (RT) role in SWL outcomes. A retrospective review was performed on 601 SWL procedures for radio-opaque stones performed by

TABLE 2.—Univariate Analysis of the Effect of RTs on SWL Outcome

RT	Mean Fluoroscopy Time (Sec) (95% CI)	Fragmentation Rate	Stone-Free Rate
A	129.0 (120.8-137.3)	82.6%	75.7%
B	158.6 (146.1-171.1)	72.5%	68.8%
C	198.3 (183.7-212.8)	72.0%	65.3%
D	168.3 (144.6-192.0)	67.2%	63.8%
E	148.4 (129.1-167.8)	68.4%	64.9%
F	170.9 (146.0-195.8)	64.6%	62.5%
P value	<.001	.004	.035

1 of 6 RTs of various experience. Follow-up outcomes were obtained with either plain films or computer tomography (CT) on 534 of the total sessions. Stone size, stone location, and the percentages of CT scans used for follow-up were statistically similar for all RTs. The outcomes evaluated were fluoroscopy time, fragmentation rate (absence of residual stone greater than 4 mm), and stone-free rate. Four urologists supervised the procedures, but no difference was found between each urologist's results.

Univariate analysis found differences in mean fluoroscopy time, fragmentation rate, and stone-free rates between the RTs (Table 2). The most experienced RT (RT A) was found to have the highest fragmentation and stone-free rate while maintaining the lowest mean fluoroscopy time. The study also presented the multivariate analysis of SWL outcomes among the 3 most experienced RTs. Multivariate analysis showed that RT A had improvements in fluoroscopy times and fragmentation rates compared with the other top 3 RTs that were statistically significant. There was no difference in final stone-free rate for the top 3 RTs.

This article introduces the impact of the RT on the fluoroscopy time and success rates of SWL procedures. The limits of the study include the retrospective nature and differences in follow-up imaging. Although multivariate analysis accounted for stone size and location, future studies could evaluate the effects of patient factors (body mass index, body habitus, and skin-to-stone distance) and stone factors (stone composition and density per Hounsfield units).

J. M. Mobley, MD

Pathogenesis of Bladder Calculi in the Presence of Urinary Stasis
Childs MA, Mynderse LA, Rangel LJ, et al (Mayo Clinic, Rochester, MN; et al)
J Urol 189:1347-1351, 2013

Purpose.—Although minimal evidence exists, bladder calculi in men with benign prostatic hyperplasia are thought to be secondary to bladder outlet obstruction induced urinary stasis. We performed a prospective, multi-institutional clinical trial to determine whether metabolic differences were present in men with and without bladder calculi undergoing surgical intervention for benign prostatic hyperplasia induced bladder outlet obstruction.

Materials and Methods.—Men who elected surgery for bladder outlet obstruction secondary to benign prostatic hyperplasia with and without bladder calculi were assessed prospectively and compared. Men without bladder calculi retained more than 150 ml urine post-void residual urine. Medical history, serum electrolytes and 24-hour urinary metabolic studies were compared.

Results.—Of the men 27 had bladder calculi and 30 did not. Bladder calculi were associated with previous renal stone disease in 36.7% of patients (11 of 30) vs 4% (2 of 27) and gout was associated in 13.3% (4 of 30) vs 0% (0 of 27) ($p < 0.01$ and 0.05, respectively). There was no observed difference in the history of other medical conditions or in serum electrolytes. Bladder calculi were associated with lower 24-hour urinary pH (median 5.9 vs 6.4, $p = 0.02$), lower 24-hour urinary magnesium (median 106 vs 167 mmol, $p = 0.01$) and increased 24-hour urinary uric acid supersaturation (median 2.2 vs 0.6, $p < 0.01$).

Conclusions.—In this comparative prospective analysis patients with bladder outlet obstruction and benign prostatic hyperplasia with bladder calculi were more likely to have a renal stone disease history, low urinary pH, low urinary magnesium and increased urinary uric acid supersaturation. These findings suggest that, like the pathogenesis of nephrolithiasis, the pathogenesis of bladder calculi is likely complex with multiple contributing lithogenic factors, including metabolic abnormalities and not just urinary stasis.

▶ In the absence of chronic infection or surgical reconstruction that includes intestinal interposition, bladder calculi are rare in developed countries. This is a report of a case control study evaluating bladder calculi in patients with benign prostatic hyperplasia undergoing elective surgery. The study is limited by small size, which may allow random variability to affect the endpoints. Table 1 in the original article shows comparable groups with the exception that statistically more men in the control group had urinary retention, and the post-void residual urine was also significantly higher in that group. Stone composition was mixed. Calcium oxalate stones were identified in 18 men, and calcium phosphate stones were present in 17. Low urine pH and uric acid supersaturation would predispose to uric acid stones. Prior urinary tract infections could increase urinary pH and lead to the formation of calcium phosphate stones. Calcium oxalate stones are harder to explain. Uric acid may act as a nidus for stone formation. Stasis may play a role in stone formation but does not appear to be the sole etiology.

D. E. Coplen, MD

Shock Wave Lithotripsy

Shock Wave Lithotripsy of Vesical Stones in Patients With Infravesical Obstruction: An Underused Noninvasive Approach
El-Halwagy S, Osman Y, Sheir KZ (Mansoura Univ, Egypt)
Urology 81:508-510, 2013

Objective.—To evaluate the effectiveness and safety of shock wave lithotripsy in the management vesical stones in patients with infravesical obstruction.

Materials and Methods.—From March 2007 to April 2010, 59 male patients with infravesical obstruction were treated using the Dornier Compact Delta II Lithotriptor for urinary bladder stones. The indications for shock wave lithotripsy included patients refusing invasive procedures or those with orthopedic malformations hindering the lithotomy position. The mean age was 61.6 ± 8.6 years (range 44-78), and the mean body mass index was 29 ± 5.1 kg/m^2 (range 20.5-45). The mean stone diameter was 26.6 ± 9.8 mm (range 12-50). All patients underwent an initial session and were re-evaluated using ultrasonography and urinary tract plain radiography at 2-week intervals.

Results.—All patients were treated in the supine position. The number of shocks ranged from 1910 to 9500. Of the 59 patients, 47 and 11 were cleared by 1 or 2 sessions, respectively; 1 patient required a third session to be cleared of stones. All patients develop mild hematuria and started to pass gravel in the first void after the shock wave lithotripsy session. All patients were rendered stone free within 6 weeks. During follow-up, only 2 male patients developed temporary acute urine retention necessitating urethral catheter fixation. Both patients had a neurologic insult.

Conclusion.—Extracorporeal shock wave lithotripsy is an effective, noninvasive approach to disintegrate vesical stones in patients with infravesical obstruction with adequate fragment clearance.

▶ The authors propose that shock wave lithotripsy is a good treatment for small bladder calculi in men. It may be less morbid than endoscopic removal, although percutaneous removal has good success and is minimally invasive. The authors say that all men had an obstructing prostate, although there are no data regarding symptom score, uroflow, and postvoid residual. Fragmentation was excellent, and only 2 men had trouble passing stone fragments despite the presence of obstructing prostates. Success was determined by ultrasound scan and KUB. The length of follow-up is not stated in the article. If very small fragments remain after lithotripsy, and the men have significant urinary stasis, then the risk of recurrent stones may be high. A randomized trial comparing shock wave lithotripsy and endoscopic (percutaneous or transurethral) removal is reasonable.

D. E. Coplen, MD

6 Transplantation

Cost-Effectiveness of Hypothermic Machine Preservation Versus Static Cold Storage in Renal Transplantation
Groen H, Moers C, Smits JM, et al (Univ of Groningen, The Netherlands; Eurotransplant International Foundation, Leiden, The Netherlands; et al)
Am J Transplant 12:1824-1830, 2012

Static cold storage (CS) is the most widely used organ preservation method for deceased donor kidney grafts but there is increasing evidence that hypothermic machine perfusion (MP) may result in better outcome after transplantation. We performed an economic evaluation of MP versus CS alongside a multicenter RCT investigating short- and long-term cost-effectiveness. Three hundred thirty-six consecutive kidney pairs were included, one of which was assigned to MP and one to CS. The economic evaluation combined the short-term results based on the empirical data from the study with a Markov model with a 10-year time horizon. Direct medical costs of hospital stay, dialysis treatment, and complications were included. Data regarding long-term survival, quality of life, and long-term costs were derived from literature. The short-term evaluation showed that MP reduced the risk of delayed graft function and graft failure at lower costs than CS. The Markov model revealed cost savings of $86 750 per life-year gained in favor of MP. The corresponding incremental cost-utility ratio was minus $496 223 per quality-adjusted life-year (QALY) gained. We conclude that life-years and QALYs can be gained while reducing costs at the same time, when kidneys are preserved by MP instead of CS.

▶ The optimal method of deceased donor kidney preservation remains unclear. Static cold storage (CS) in organ preservation solution has been the primary method of organ storage during the period from organ procurement to transplantation. A recent large, randomized, prospective trial suggested superiority of machine perfusion (MP) over CS, as MP-preserved kidneys had a reduced risk of delayed graft function (DGF) and improved 1-year graft survival.[1] Although this and other studies have found a clinical benefit of MP over CS, the economic impact continues to be an obstacle. MP is more labor intensive, as it requires specialized equipment and personnel, which presumably increase the cost.

This study utilized outcomes from the previous randomized trial to model cost effectiveness of MP versus CS in renal transplantation. From both a short- and long-term perspective, the model suggests that MP may substantially reduce the costs of deceased donor kidney transplantation compared with CS. These cost savings are modeled to occur largely through the improved graft survival and lower DGF rates with MP-preserved kidneys. The costs of short- and/or long-term dialysis, which become necessary when the graft does not function, seem to markedly outweigh the up front costs of MP.

V. Krishnamurthi, MD

Reference

1. Moers C, Smits JM, Maathuis MD, et al. Machine perfusion or cold storage in deceased-donor kidney transplantation. *N Engl J Med.* 2009;360:7-19.

7 Trauma

High-grade renal injury: non-operative management of urinary extravasation and prediction of long-term outcomes
Long J-A, Fiard G, Descotes J-L, et al (Grenoble Univ Hosp, France)
BJU Int 111:E249-E255, 2013

Objective.—• To predict the outcomes of a non-operative approach to managing urinary extravasation after blunt renal trauma.

Patients and Methods.—• A prospective observational study was conducted between January 2004 and October 2011. First-line non-operative management was proposed for 99 patients presenting with a grade IV blunt renal injury according to the revised American Association for the Surgery of Trauma (AAST) classification. Among them, 72 patients presented with a urinary extravasation.

• Management and outcomes were recorded and compared between patients presenting and those who did not present with urinary leakage. Relative postoperative renal function was assessed 6 months after the trauma using dimercapto-succinic acid renal scintigraphy.

• Predictors of the need for endoscopic or surgical management and long-term renal function were evaluated on multivariate analysis.

Results —• Among patients with urinary leakage, endoscopic ureteric stent placement and open surgery were required in 37% and 1.5%, respectively.

• On multivariate analysis, fever of >38.5°C and ureteric clot obstruction were independent predictors of the need for ureteric stent placement. The only predictor of open surgery was the percentage of devitalised parenchyma.

• Long-term renal function loss was correlated to the percentage of devitalised parenchyma and associated visceral lesions. Urinary extravasation did not predict surgical intervention or long-term renal function loss.

Conclusions.—• Urinary extravasation after blunt renal trauma can be successfully managed conservatively and does not predict long-term decreased renal function or surgery requirement.

• A devascularised parenchyma volume of >25% predicts a higher rate of surgery and poorer renal function.

Study Type.—Therapy (outcomes).

Level of Evidence.—2b.

What's Known on the Subject? and What Does the Study Add?.—High-grade renal trauma seems to be eligible for conservative management. Ureteric stent placement raises issues about its usefulness and its timing. Predictive factors of post-trauma function and surgery need to be known.

Urinary extravasation is not associated with poor functional outcome. Ureteric stenting is needed only in case of sepsis and ureteric clot retention. The only independent predictor of long-term renal function is the importance of devascularised renal fragments.

▶ Conservative management of high-grade renal trauma is the standard. The availability of competent interventional radiologists for angioembolization decreases the need for surgical exploration for hemorrhage. The authors attempt to address whether a ureteral stent should be placed for urinary extravasation, but the variability in patient characteristics and indications for stent placement preclude any definitive conclusions. In general, patients with extravasation did well without a stent. A stent may actually be obstructive and cause more harm than good. In the absence of sepsis or uretero-pelvic junction disruption, extravasation should be observed.

D. E. Coplen, MD

8 Female Urology

Diagnostics

A randomized trial of urodynamic testing before stress-incontinence surgery
Nager CW, Urinary Incontinence Treatment Network (Univ of California at San Diego, La Julla; et al)
N Engl J Med 366:1987-1997, 2012

Background.—Urodynamic studies are commonly performed in women before surgery for stress urinary incontinence, but there is no good evidence that they improve outcomes.

Methods.—We performed a multicenter, randomized, noninferiority trial involving women with uncomplicated, demonstrable stress urinary incontinence to compare outcomes after preoperative office evaluation and urodynamic tests or evaluation only. The primary outcome was treatment success at 12 months, defined as a reduction in the score on the Urogenital Distress Inventory of 70% or more and a response of "much better" or "very much better" on the Patient Global Impression of Improvement. The predetermined noninferiority margin was 11 percentage points.

Results.—A total of 630 women were randomly assigned to undergo office evaluation with urodynamic tests or evaluation only (315 per group); the proportion in whom treatment was successful was 76.9% in the urodynamic-testing group versus 77.2% in the evaluation-only group (difference, −0.3 percentage points; 95% confidence interval, −7.5 to 6.9), which was consistent with noninferiority. There were no significant between-group differences in secondary measures of incontinence severity, quality of life, patient satisfaction, rates of positive provocative stress tests, voiding dysfunction, or adverse events. Women who underwent urodynamic tests were significantly less likely to receive a diagnosis of overactive bladder and more likely to receive a diagnosis of voiding-phase dysfunction, but these changes did not lead to significant between-group differences in treatment selection or outcomes.

Conclusions.—For women with uncomplicated, demonstrable stress urinary incontinence, preoperative office evaluation alone was not inferior to evaluation with urodynamic testing for outcomes at 1 year. (Funded by the National Institute of Diabetes and Digestive and Kidney Diseases and the Eunice Kennedy Shriver National Institute of Child Health and Human Development; ClinicalTrials.gov number, NCT00803959.)

▶ This multicenter randomized trial compared the outcomes of stress urinary incontinence surgery in patients undergoing preoperative invasive urodynamics versus those not undergoing such diagnostic testing. This is important information as the value of such testing has been questioned because it is expensive, invasive, and carries with it potential morbidity including infection, dysuria, and hematuria. In this highly selected group of patients, performance of urodynamic testing was not associated with better outcomes. However, all of the patients randomized in this study had complaints of pure stress urinary incontinence (SUI) or stress-predominant mixed incontinence and demonstrated SUI on physical examination. Furthermore, patients with neurogenic disease, history of prior lower urinary tract surgery, or radiation therapy were excluded. Whether such findings are generalizable to a more complex group of patients is unclear. Notably, more than 4000 patients were screened to get the population under study, suggesting that these were indeed highly selected patients.

E. S. Rovner, MD

5-Year Continence Rates, Satisfaction and Adverse Events of Burch Urethropexy and Fascial Sling Surgery for Urinary Incontinence

Brubaker L, for the Urinary Incontinence Treatment Network (Loyola Univ Chicago, IL; et al)
J Urol 187:1324-1330, 2012

Purpose.—We characterized continence, satisfaction and adverse events in women at least 5 years after Burch urethropexy or fascial sling with longitudinal followup of randomized clinical trial participants.

Materials and Methods.—Of 655 women who participated in a randomized surgical trial comparing the efficacy of the Burch and sling treatments 482 (73.6%) enrolled in this long-term observational study. Urinary continence status was assessed yearly for a minimum of 5 years postoperatively. Continence was defined as no urinary leakage on a 3-day voiding diary, and no self-reported stress incontinence symptoms and no stress incontinence surgical re-treatment.

Results.—Incontinent participants were more likely to enroll in the followup study than continent patients (85.5% vs 52.2%) regardless of surgical group ($p<0.0001$). Overall the continence rates were lower in the Burch urethropexy group than in the fascial sling group ($p = 0.002$). The continence rates at 5 years were 24.1% (95% CI 18.5 to 29.7) vs 30.8% (95% CI 24.7 to 36.9), respectively. Satisfaction at 5 years was related to continence status and was higher in women undergoing sling surgery (83% vs 73%, $p = 0.04$). Satisfaction decreased with time ($p = 0.001$) and remained higher in the sling group ($p = 0.03$). The 2 groups had similar adverse event rates (Burch 10% vs sling 9%) and similar numbers of participants with adverse events (Burch 23 vs sling 22).

Conclusions.—Continence rates in both groups decreased substantially during 5 years, yet most women reported satisfaction with their continence status. Satisfaction was higher in continent women and in those who underwent fascial sling surgery, despite the voiding dysfunction associated with this procedure.

▶ These authors are to be congratulated on following this subset of patients from the SISTEr trial for an extended period. It is noteworthy and rare for a cohort to be followed so assiduously from such a high-quality randomized control trial for stress urinary incontinence. Though the continence rates fall off precipitously, and almost embarrassingly so, patient satisfaction rates remain reasonable. Is this the best we can expect from our surgeries for stress incontinence at 5 years? Both of the surgeries performed in this trial are not commonly performed these days in the era of the midurethral polypropylene sling. However, given the medico-legal issues currently confronting vaginal mesh, it would not be beyond possibility that if the meshes are withdrawn from the marketplace, we will be back to performing such surgeries with more regularity.

E. S. Rovner, MD

A Midurethral Sling to Reduce Incontinence after Vaginal Prolapse Repair
Wei JT, for the Pelvic Floor Disorders Network (Univ of Michigan, Ann Arbor; et al)
N Engl J Med 366:2358-2367, 2012

Background.—Women without stress urinary incontinence undergoing vaginal surgery for pelvic-organ prolapse are at risk for postoperative urinary incontinence. A midurethral sling may be placed at the time of prolapse repair to reduce this risk.

Methods.—We performed a multicenter trial involving women without symptoms of stress incontinence and with anterior prolapse (of stage 2 or higher on a Pelvic Organ Prolapse Quantification system examination) who were planning to undergo vaginal prolapse surgery. Women were randomly assigned to receive either a midurethral sling or sham incisions during surgery. One primary end point was urinary incontinence or treatment for this condition at 3 months. The second primary end point was the presence of incontinence at 12 months, allowing for subsequent treatment for incontinence.

Results.—Of the 337 women who underwent randomization, 327 (97%) completed follow-up at 1 year. At 3 months, the rate of urinary incontinence (or treatment) was 23.6% in the sling group and 49.4% in the sham group ($P < 0.001$). At 12 months, urinary incontinence (allowing for subsequent treatment of incontinence) was present in 27.3% and 43.0% of patients in the sling and sham groups, respectively ($P = 0.002$). The number needed to treat with a sling to prevent one case of urinary incontinence at 12 months was 6.3. The rate of bladder perforation was higher in the sling group than in the sham group (6.7% vs. 0%), as were rates of urinary tract infection (31.0% vs. 18.3%), major bleeding complications (3.1% vs. 0%), and incomplete bladder emptying 6 weeks after surgery (3.7% vs. 0%) ($P \leq 0.05$ for all comparisons).

Conclusions.—A prophylactic midurethral sling inserted during vaginal prolapse surgery resulted in a lower rate of urinary incontinence at 3 and 12 months but higher rates of adverse events. (Funded by the Eunice Kennedy Shriver National Institute of Child Health and Human Development and the National Institutes of Health Office of Research on Women's Health; OPUS ClinicalTrials.gov number, NCT00460434.)

► This is a well-done randomized and well-controlled (via sham) trial demonstrating the beneficial effects on reducing the incidence of postoperative stress urinary incontinence by placing a transvaginal sling at the time of transvaginal prolapse surgery. These results mirror the findings of the CARE trial published several years ago in which abdominal Burch colposuspension was shown to be beneficial in patients undergoing transabdominal prolapse repair. Complications of additional surgery, such as a sling in this setting, should always be weighed against the potential benefits, and in this trial the complications attributed to the additional surgery were minimal. Of course, surgical success and the risk of complications are somewhat dependent on surgical expertise, experience, and patient selection. Thus, each individual surgeon must determine whether the risk of additional surgery in *preventing* postoperative stress urinary incontinence is worth the potential risk of additional complications related to the surgery based on their own clinical experience.

E. S. Rovner, MD

Symptoms and Risk Factors Associated with First Urinary Tract Infection in College Age Women: A Prospective Cohort Study

Vincent CR, Thomas TL, Reyes L, et al (Univ of Florida, Gainesville)
J Urol 189:904-910, 2013

Purpose.—We identified epidemiological risk factors for the initial urinary tract infection in females of college age compared to age matched controls.

Materials and Methods.—We performed a prospective cohort study from July 2001 to January 2006 at the student health care facility at our institution. A total of 180 women experiencing a first urinary tract infection were compared to 80 asymptomatic women with no urinary tract infection history who served as controls. Urinalysis and urine culture were done at study enrollment. Questionnaires were used to obtain information on clinical symptoms and behaviors, including sexual and dietary practices, and alcohol consumption. Logistic regression was performed to identify potential risk factors in women who presented with an initial urinary tract infection compared with controls. Principal component analysis was then done to identify key sexual activity variables for multiple regression models.

Results.—Urinary frequency and urgency were the most common urinary tract infection symptoms. Recent sexual activity was a significant risk factor for urinary tract infection with vaginal intercourse ($p = 0.002$) and the number of sexual partners in the last 2 weeks ($p < 0.001$) as the 2 primary variables. Alcohol consumption was associated with 2 of the 3 main principal components of sexual activity. Caffeinated beverage consumption also increased the risk of urinary tract infection ($p < 0.04$). Escherichia coli was the predominant pathogen isolated, followed by urease positive microbes.

Conclusions.—Recent sexual activity, the frequency of that activity and the number of sexual partners pose an increased risk of urinary tract infection. Alcohol consumption frequency and amount correlated with these behaviors.

▶ Recurrent urinary tract infections (UTIs) are a major source of morbidity in outpatient urology practice. Much has been written in the lay and professional literature regarding the risk factors for acquiring UTIs in the community. Much of what has been written and promulgated over the years, especially in the lay literature, is not supported by scientific literature. This study supports prior work in the area suggesting that increased sexual activity and partners are associated with increased risk of UTI. Notably, this was a young healthy cohort of sexually active ambulatory college-age women. Thus, these findings are not generalizable to the entire population of those with recurrent UTIs, which represents a diverse population, including those with voiding dysfunction, genitourinary anatomic and physiologic abnormalities, and comorbid medical illnesses. Of course, what remains is the question of what (other than abstinence) is the optimal method of preventing such infections in this population?

E. S. Rovner, MD

Pharmacologic Therapy

Anticholinergic Therapy vs. OnabotulinumtoxinA for Urgency Urinary Incontinence

Visco AG, for the Pelvic Floor Disorders Network (Duke Univ Med Ctr, Durham, NC; et al)
N Engl J Med 367:1803-1813, 2012

Background.—Anticholinergic medications and onabotulinumtoxinA are used to treat urgency urinary incontinence, but data directly comparing the two types of therapy are needed.

Methods.—We performed a double-blind, double-placebo—controlled, randomized trial involving women with idiopathic urgency urinary incontinence who had five or more episodes of urgency urinary incontinence per 3-day period, as recorded in a diary. For a 6-month period, participants were randomly assigned to daily oral anticholinergic medication (solifenacin, 5 mg initially, with possible escalation to 10 mg and, if necessary, subsequent switch to trospium XR, 60 mg) plus one intradetrusor injection of saline or one intradetrusor injection of 100 U of onabotulinumtoxinA plus daily oral placebo. The primary outcome was the reduction from baseline in mean episodes of urgency urinary incontinence per day over the 6-month period, as recorded in 3-day diaries submitted monthly. Secondary outcomes included complete resolution of urgency urinary incontinence, quality of life, use of catheters, and adverse events.

Results.—Of 249 women who underwent randomization, 247 were treated, and 241 had data available for the primary outcome analyses. The mean reduction in episodes of urgency urinary incontinence per day over the course of 6 months, from a baseline average of 5.0 per day, was 3.4 in the anticholinergic group and 3.3 in the onabotulinumtoxinA group ($P = 0.81$). Complete resolution of urgency urinary incontinence was reported by 13% and 27% of the women, respectively ($P = 0.003$). Quality of life improved in both groups, without significant between-group differences. The anticholinergic group had a higher rate of dry mouth (46% vs. 31%, $P = 0.02$) but lower rates of catheter use at 2 months (0% vs. 5%, $P = 0.01$) and urinary tract infections (13% vs. 33%, $P < 0.001$).

Conclusions.—Oral anticholinergic therapy and onabotulinumtoxinA by injection were associated with similar reductions in the frequency of daily episodes of urgency urinary incontinence. The group receiving onabotulinumtoxinA was less likely to have dry mouth and more likely to have complete resolution of urgency urinary incontinence but had higher rates of transient urinary retention and urinary tract infections. (Funded by the Eunice Kennedy Shriver National Institute of Child Health and Human Development and the National Institutes of Health Office of Research on Women's Health; ClinicalTrials.gov number, NCT01166438.)

▶ The results from this well-done randomized placebo controlled trial suggest some degree of equivalence between intravesical OnabotulinumtoxinA (BOT) and antimuscarinic (AMT) therapy for the reduction of urinary incontinence episodes at 6 months in affected individuals. These findings were independent of the baseline number of incontinence episodes or prior drug therapy. Dry rates favored BOT but were rather low in both groups as measured by a 3-day diary. Adverse events attributable to each therapy were as expected (AMT produced more dry mouth than BOT, but BOT was associated with more urinary retention than AMT). It is important to note that this study protocol was not necessarily reflective of clinical practice. BOT is considered a third-line therapy for those patients with overactive bladder failing pharmacological therapy. Approximately 60% of patients in this trial had not received prior drug therapy. In addition, of the approximately 40% of patients who had received prior drug therapy, all washed out from their therapy before entry into the study and it is possible that some of these individuals who washed out were doing fine on their drug therapy. Both of these factors may have enriched the response rates seen in this trial. Finally, these results should not be extrapolated to the "dry" overactive bladder population because such individuals were not studied. An interesting finding of this study was that at 1 and 6 months after discontinuing drug therapy, approximately 50% and 25% of patients still had adequate control of their symptoms. Such findings cannot be explained by pharmacological effects of the discontinued drug, but they are noteworthy nonetheless.

E. S. Rovner, MD

Reconstruction

Long-Term Results of Artificial Urinary Sphincter for Women with Type III Stress Urinary Incontinence

Costa P, Poinas G, Ben Naoum K, et al (Montpellier Université I, Nîmes, France)
Eur Urol 63:753-758, 2013

Background.—The use of the artificial urinary sphincter (AUS) in women is limited.

Objective.—To analyse long-term results and mechanical survival of the AUS (AMS 800; American Medical Systems, Minnetonka, MN, USA) in women with stress urinary incontinence (SUI) due to intrinsic sphincter deficiency (ISD).

Design, Setting, and Participants.—Women with SUI who were treated between January 1987 and March 2007 were included in this prospective study. Only women with low closure pressure at urethral profile and negative continence tests, indicators of severe ISD, were included.

Interventions.—An AUS was implanted. The surgical technique was modified in 1999, involving opening the endopelvic fascia on both sides and dissection in contact with the vaginal wall.

Outcome Measurements and Statistical Analysis.—Assessment of complications was made pre- and postoperatively and continence status was based on pad usage. Kaplan-Meier survival curves were used to calculate mechanical survival of the device. Student t test and the chi-square test were used to compare continence and complication rates.

Results and Limitations.—A total of 376 AUS were implanted in 344 patients, whose mean age was 57 yr. The mean follow-up, plus or minus standard deviation, was 9.6 ± 4.0 yr. At last follow-up, postoperative continence rates, assessed as fully continent (no leakage), socially incontinent (some drops but no pad), or incontinent (one pad or more), were 85.6%, 8.8%, and 5.6%, respectively. The 3-, 5-, and 10-yr device survival rates were 92.0%, 88.6%, and 69.2%, respectively. The mean mechanical survival was 176 mo (14.7 yr). Three risk factors for AUS survival were the number of previous incontinence surgeries, the presence of neurogenic bladder, and simultaneous augmentation enterocystoplasty. Principal limitation of the study is the absence of validated incontinence questionnaire.

Conclusions.—The AUS provides excellent outcome in women with ISD, with low explantation rate and very good device survival.

▶ This prospective study represents the largest series of women implanted with an artificial urinary sphincter (AUS) and has the longest follow-up (mean, 9.6 years). Although the use of AUS in women is limited, in this study, 376

AUSs were implanted over a 20-year period in women with low-closure pressure at the urethral profile or intrinsic sphincter deficiency (ISD)/type III stress urinary incontinence, and the long-term results/mechanical device survival were investigated. At last follow-up, 85.6% were fully continent, whereas 8.8% had social continence and 5.6% required one pad or more. Three-, 5-, and 10-year device survival rates were 92%, 88.6%, and 69.2%, respectively. The mean mechanical survival was 14.7 years. This represented very good outcomes in nonneurogenic bladder patients and good device survival in the setting of a low explantation rate.

This study discusses an alternative to more commonly performed sling procedures, particularly in patients with severe ISD, and a fixed/nonhypermobile urethra in which success rates for transvaginal tape have been reported as low as 17%. A total of 46.5% of patients had a prior Burch colposuspension. An enterocystoplasty was performed at the same time as AUS in patients with poor compliance/neurogenic bladder and ISD. De novo bladder overactivity occurred in 9.8% of patients. Although it is the gold standard for male urinary sphincter incompetence, only 1% of women with incontinence are implanted with an AUS.

Of note, in 1999, a technical modification to the procedure, including incision of the endopelvic fascia on both sides of the proximal urethra, was introduced, which minimized blind passage. Before this, 8.8% of patients had a urethral injury, and 6.7% had vaginal opening (which can be managed conservatively with postoperative vaginal antibiotic packing), whereas after 1999, these complications decreased to 1.7% each. A total of 12.8% of implants had nonmechanical complications (acute retention/infection/erosion) leading to AUS removal. A total of 13.6% of implants had mechanical complications, leading to partial revision in 5.9% or complete revision in 7.7%.

This procedure is a potential alternative to bladder suspension/sling procedures. With the pump located in the labia majora, patients need to have the comfort level, hand strength, and coordination to manipulate the device. Although it has gained increased popularity in a complex subset of patients with severe ISD and a fixed urethra, it requires good patient tissue quality and is certainly more technically challenging and more expensive and carries the concern of mechanical device failure compared with alternative therapies, such as suburethral slings and bulking agents.

E. S. Rovner, MD

Autologous Muscle Derived Cell Therapy for Stress Urinary Incontinence: A Prospective, Dose Ranging Study

Carr LK, Robert M, Kultgen PL, et al (Sunnybrook Health Sciences Centre, Toronto, Ontario, Canada; Univ of Calgary, Alberta, Canada; MED Inst, Inc, West Lafayette, IN; et al)
J Urol 189:595-601, 2013

Purpose.—In this feasibility study we assessed the 12-month safety and potential efficacy of autologous muscle derived cells (Cook MyoSite

Incorporated, Pittsburgh, Pennsylvania) as therapy for stress urinary incontinence.

Materials and Methods.—A total of 38 women in whom stress urinary incontinence had not improved with conservative therapy for 12 or more months underwent intrasphincter injection of low doses (1, 2, 4, 8 or 16×10^6) or high doses (32, 64 or 128×10^6) of autologous muscle derived cells, which were derived from biopsies of their quadriceps femoris. All patients could elect a second treatment of the same dose after 3-month followup. Assessments were made at 1, 3, 6 and 12 months after the last treatment. The primary end point was the incidence and severity of adverse events. In addition, changes in stress urinary incontinence severity were evaluated by pad test, diary of incontinence episodes and quality of life surveys.

Results.—Of the 38 patients 33 completed the study. Treatment related complications were limited to minor events such as pain/bruising at the biopsy and injection sites. Of patients who received 2 treatments of autologous muscle derived cells who were eligible for analysis, a higher percentage of those in the high dose vs the low dose group experienced a 50% or greater reduction in pad weight (88.9%, 8 of 9 vs 61.5%, 8 of 13), had a 50% or greater reduction in diary reported stress leaks (77.8%, 7 of 9 vs 53.3%, 8 of 15) and had 0 to 1 leaks during 3 days (88.9%, 8 of 9 vs 33.3%, 5 of 15) at final followup.

Conclusions.—Injection of autologous muscle derived cells in a wide range of doses appears safe with no major treatment related adverse events reported. In addition, treatment with autologous muscle derived cells shows promise for relieving stress urinary incontinence symptoms and improving quality of life.

▶ This is a small feasibility and safety study without a control arm and thus has substantial limitations. Nonetheless, the modest improvements seen in these patients especially at the higher doses are intriguing. Follow up in this study is relatively short, given the chronic nature of stress urinary incontinence and the known short-term efficacy of virtually all injectable bulking agents. The longer term data should allow differentiation between this injectable therapy and the existing bulking agents that often fail in the long term. Additionally, given the alternative treatments currently available for stress urinary incontinence, including the midurethral sling, which are safe and effective, the efficacy "bar" is set fairly high.

E. S. Rovner, MD

9 Benign Prostatic Hyperplasia

Epidemiology and Biomarkers

Urodynamic Effects of Transrectal Intraprostatic *Ona botulinum* Toxin A Injections for Symptomatic Benign Prostatic Hyperplasia

de Kort LMO, Kok ET, Jonges TN, et al (Univ Med Ctr Utrecht, the Netherlands)
Urology 80:889-893, 2012

Objective.—To investigate urodynamic, symptomatic, and histologic effects of intraprostatic injection with *Ona botulinum* toxin A for benign prostatic hyperplasia.

Methods.—Patients > 55 years with symptomatic benign prostatic hyperplasia failing medical therapy were treated. Inclusion criteria were International Prostate Symptom Score > 7, prostate volume 30-50 cm^3, and urodynamic bladder outlet obstruction > Schäfer grade 2. A transrectal intraprostatic injection of 200 IU *Ona botulinum* toxin A was given. Filling cystometry and pressure flow studies were performed at 3, 6, and 12 months post injection. International Prostate Symptom Score, International Prostate Symptom Score quality of life, prostate-specific antigen, and prostate volume were measured up until 12 months; prostate biopsies before and after *Ona botulinum* toxin A injection were done for histology and cell proliferation.

Results.—Fifteen men (mean age 64.9 years) were included. *Ona botulinum* toxin A injection was well tolerated with few complications. Postvoid residual improved (170 to 80 mL), but maximum flow rate and bladder outlet resistance parameters did not change during follow-up. International Prostate Symptom Score and International Prostate Symptom Score quality of life improved (22 to 13 and 5 to 2, respectively), whereas prostate-specific antigen and prostate volume remained unaltered. Cell proliferation did not decrease and in 37% and 64% of pre- and posttreatment biopsies, respectively, some degree of prostatitis was found. Ten of 15 patients eventually underwent transurethral prostate resection because of persisting symptoms.

Conclusion.—Intraprostatic *Ona botulinum* toxin A for symptomatic benign prostatic hyperplasia did not affect urodynamic outcomes, except for postvoid residual. Although symptom scores improved, we were not

37

able to show change in prostate volume, prostate-specific antigen, or histologic outcomes. A placebo effect of intraprostatic *Ona botulinum* toxin A could not be ruled out.

▶ This article reports the urodynamic outcomes of a trial involving intraprostatic injection of *Ona botulinum* toxin A for the treatment of benign prostatic hyperplasia (BPH). This was a small trial in a highly selected group of patients. Bladder injection was not performed in this trial, and *Ona botulinum* toxin A is not indicated for the treatment of BPH in the United States.

It is noteworthy in this trial that symptoms improved, but urodynamic parameters did not except for postvoid residual (PVR). Such findings are not inconsistent with the data published for most oral pharmacotherapy (α-blockers and 5-α-reductase inhibitors) in which symptom improvement is greater than urodynamic improvement (in such drug trials, uroflow, not PVR, were checked). What is the mechanism for symptom improvement in these patients without urodynamic improvement? It is not clear. The authors attributed it to a placebo effect, and, although this may be true, there may be other explanations as well, including an unexplained local afferent/efferent effect in the prostate. It would be interesting to see what the outcomes were for the patients who underwent transurethral resection of the prostate after not responding to this injection.

E. S. Rovner, MD

Surgical Treatment

Effects of bipolar and monopolar transurethral resection of the prostate on urinary and erectile function: a prospective randomized comparative study

Akman T, Binbay M, Tekinarslan E, et al (Bezmialem Vakif Univ, Istanbul, Turkey; Haseki Training and Res Hosp, Istanbul, Turkey)
BJU Int 111:129-136, 2013

Objective.—• To evaluate the outcomes of bipolar vs conventional monopolar transurethral resection of the prostate (TURP) on urinary and erectile function.

Material and Methods.—• A total of 286 patients with benign prostatic hyperplasia (BPH) were randomized to bipolar or monopolar conventional TURP treatment groups.

• Operative and early postoperative variables and complications were recorded and all patients were re-evaluated at 1, 3, 6 and 12 months after surgery using the International Prostate Symptom Score (IPSS), uroflowmetry, post-void residual urine volume (PVR) and the erectile function domain of the International Index of Erectile Function (IIEF-ED).

• A comparative evaluation of erectile function was performed on 188 preoperatively non-catheterized patients with regular sexual partners.

Results.—• The operating time was shorter in the bipolar TURP group. Postoperative bleeding and blood transfusion requirements did not significantly differ between the two groups. Sodium levels were significantly lower in the monopolar group than in the bipolar group.

• Transuretheral resection syndrome developed in two (1.4%) patients in the monopolar group. Both groups had similar and significantly improved IPSS values, maximum urinary flow rate values and PVR measurement.

• ED worsened in 32 (17.0%) patients, improved in 53 (28.2%) patients, and was unchanged in 103 (54.8%) patients. Changes in the IIEF scores during the follow-up period were similar between the bipolar and monopolar groups.

Conclusion.—• Bipolar TURP is a safe and effective procedure that is associated with a significantly shorter operating time, a smaller reduction in serum sodium levels and a similar efficacy compared with conventional monopolar TURP.

▶ This very relevant randomized study compares the use of monopolar and bipolar energy for transurethral resection of the prostate (TURP). This study is particularly robust in that the decision on energy source was made by randomization, thus producing a well-matched population at baseline, with respect to the subjects themselves and the timing of their procedures.

Functional urination outcomes were similar between groups. The rate of complications was similar between groups although TURP syndrome occurred in 2 patients from the monopolar group and none from the bipolar group. There was no difference in sexual function outcome as assessed by the International Index of Erectile Function (IIEF) between the 2 energy sources.

These data demonstrate that bipolar energy is equivalent or superior to monopolar energy for TURP in most safety endpoints, including sexual function outcomes. The net rate of change in erectile function is also of interest to practicing clinicians; these data may represent approximate estimates of likelihood in change of erectile function after TURP for benign prostatic hyperplasia. Unfortunately, the authors report that no parameter (pre- or postoperative) was predictive of change in IIEF scores, so specific prognostication of erectile function outcome post-TURP based on patient characteristics does not appear possible from these data.

A. W. Shindel, MD

Medical Treatment

Prospective, Randomized, Double-Blind, Vehicle Controlled, Multicenter Phase IIb Clinical Trial of the Pore Forming Protein PRX302 for Targeted Treatment of Symptomatic Benign Prostatic Hyperplasia

Elhilali MM, Pommerville P, Yocum RC, et al (McGill Univ, Montreal, Quebec, Canada; Can-Med Clinical Res, Victoria, British Columbia, Canada; Sophiris Bio Corp., La Jolla, CA; et al)

J Urol 189:1421-1426, 2013

Purpose.—We conducted a safety and efficacy evaluation of intraprostatic injection of PRX302, a modified pore forming protein (proaerolysin) activated by prostate specific antigen, as a highly targeted, localized approach to treat lower urinary tract symptoms due to benign prostatic hyperplasia.

Materials and Methods.—A total of 92 patients with I-PSS (International Prostate Symptom Score) 15 or greater, peak urine flow 12 ml or less per second and prostate volume 30 to 100 ml were randomized 2:1 to a single ultrasound guided intraprostatic injection of PRX302 vs vehicle (placebo) in this phase IIb double-blind study. Injection was 20% of prostate volume and 0.6 μg PRX302 per gm prostate. Peak urine flow was determined by a blinded reviewer. Benign prostatic hyperplasia medications were prohibited. The primary data set of efficacy evaluable patients (73) was analyzed using last observation carried forward.

Results.—PRX302 treatment resulted in an approximate 9-point reduction in I-PSS and 3 ml per second increase in peak urine flow that were statistically significant changes from baseline compared to vehicle. Efficacy was sustained for 12 months. Early withdrawal for other benign prostatic hyperplasia treatment was more common for patients in the vehicle group. Relative to vehicle, PRX302 apparent toxicity was mild, transient, and limited to local discomfort/pain and irritative urinary symptoms occurring in the first few days, with no effect on erectile function.

Conclusions.—A single administration of PRX302 as a short, outpatient based procedure was well tolerated in patients with lower urinary tract symptoms due to benign prostatic hyperplasia. PRX302 produced clinically meaningful and statistically significant improvement in patient subjective (I-PSS) and quantitative objective (peak urine flow) measures sustained for 12 months. The side effect profile is favorable with most effects attributed to the injection itself and not related to drug toxicity.

▶ The authors evaluate the efficacy of an intraprostatic injection of a genetically modified protein that is activated only by intraprostatic prostate-specific antigen and causes cell death. In theory, this is a highly targeted local therapy that would potentially avoid the side effects of oral and surgical treatments for benign prostatic hyperplasia. There was statistically significant improvement in both flow rate and International Prostate Symptom Score (IPSS), but the clinical significance, for example, of a flow rate of 12 mL/s vs 10 mL/s after treatment is unclear. In fact, at 350 days, there was not a statistical difference between the IPSS between the treatment and placebo groups. Fig 2 in the original article shows the significant placebo effect in these types of studies and drives home the absolute importance of double-blind randomization in these studies.

D. E. Coplen, MD

10 Male Incontinence/ Voiding Dysfunction

Impact of Complete Bladder Neck Preservation on Urinary Continence, Quality of Life and Surgical Margins After Radical Prostatectomy: A Randomized, Controlled, Single Blind Trial
Nyarangi-Dix JN, Radtke JP, Hadaschik B, et al (Univ of Hoidelberg, Germany)
J Urol 189:891-898, 2013

Purpose.—We investigated the influence of bladder neck preservation on urinary continence, quality of life and surgical margins after radical prostatectomy.

Materials and Methods.—A total of 208 men who presented for radical prostatectomy were randomized to complete bladder neck preservation with subsequent urethro-urethral anastomosis or to no preservation as controls. Patients with failed bladder neck preservation were not included in study. We documented objective continence by the 24-hour pad test, social continence by the number of pads per day and quality of life outcomes by the validated Incontinence Quality of Life questionnaire in a single blind setting. Cancer resection was assessed by surgical margin status.

Results.—At 0, 3, 6 and 12 months mean urine loss in the control vs the bladder neck preservation group was 713.3 vs 237.0, 49.6 vs 15.6, 44.4 vs 5.5 and 25.4 vs 3.1 gm, respectively (each $p < 0.001$). At 3, 6 and 12 months in the control vs the preservation group the social continence rate was 55.3% vs 84.2% ($p < 0.001$), 74.8% vs 89.5% ($p = 0.05$) and 81.4% vs 94.7% ($p = 0.027$), and the quality of life score was 80.4 vs 90.3 ($p < 0.001$), 85.4 vs 91.7 ($p = 0.016$) and 86.0 vs 93.8 ($p < 0.001$), respectively. We noted significantly less urine loss, higher objective and social continence rates, and higher quality of life scores after complete bladder neck preservation at all followup points. On multiple logistic regression analysis complete bladder neck preservation was an independent positive predictor of continence. No significant difference was found in surgical margin status between the control and bladder neck preservation groups (12.5% vs 14.7%, $p = 0.65$).

Conclusions.—In what is to our knowledge the first prospective, randomized, controlled, single blind trial complete bladder neck preservation during radical prostatectomy was associated with a significantly higher urinary continence rate and increased patient satisfaction without compromising resection margins.

▶ Despite advances in surgical techniques for surgical extirpation of the prostate for prostate cancer, including minimally invasive techniques such as laparoscopy and robotics, postoperative complications, such as stress urinary incontinence, remain problematic in many patients. Many variations in surgical technique have been described in open radical prostatectomy as well as minimally invasive techniques to reduce the incidence of postoperative urinary stress incontinence. Such variations include, but are not limited to, preservation of the puboprostatic ligaments, cavernosal nerve-identifying and sparing techniques, sural nerve grafting, variations in incision and dissection of the lateral prostatic fascia and Denonvilliers fascia, reconstruction of the posterior rhabdosphincter, and bladder neck sparing. This article, describing a bladder neck—sparing technique, is the first such operative variation to be subjected to the rigor of a randomized, controlled trial. Importantly, this technique did not compromise cancer control.

E. S. Rovner, MD

Long-Term Functional Outcomes after Treatment for Localized Prostate Cancer

Resnick MJ, Koyama T, Fan K-H, et al (Vanderbilt Univ, Nashville, TN; et al)
N Engl J Med 368:436-445, 2013

Background.—The purpose of this analysis was to compare long-term urinary, bowel, and sexual function after radical prostatectomy or external-beam radiation therapy.

Methods.—The Prostate Cancer Outcomes Study (PCOS) enrolled 3533 men in whom prostate cancer had been diagnosed in 1994 or 1995. The current cohort comprised 1655 men in whom localized prostate cancer had been diagnosed between the ages of 55 and 74 years and who had undergone either surgery (1164 men) or radiotherapy (491 men). Functional status was assessed at baseline and at 2, 5, and 15 years after diagnosis. We used multivariable propensity scoring to compare functional outcomes according to treatment.

Results.—Patients undergoing prostatectomy were more likely to have urinary incontinence than were those undergoing radiotherapy at 2 years (odds ratio, 6.22; 95% confidence interval [CI], 1.92 to 20.29) and 5 years (odds ratio, 5.10; 95% CI, 2.29 to 11.36). However, no significant between-group difference in the odds of urinary incontinence was noted at 15 years. Similarly, although patients undergoing prostatectomy were more likely to have erectile dysfunction at 2 years (odds ratio, 3.46; 95% CI, 1.93 to 6.17) and 5 years (odds ratio, 1.96; 95% CI, 1.05 to 3.63), no significant between-group difference was noted at 15 years. Patients undergoing prostatectomy were less likely to have bowel urgency at 2 years (odds ratio, 0.39; 95% CI, 0.22 to 0.68) and 5 years (odds ratio,

0.47; 95% CI, 0.26 to 0.84), again with no significant between-group difference in the odds of bowel urgency at 15 years.

Conclusions.—At 15 years, no significant relative differences in disease-specific functional outcomes were observed among men undergoing prostatectomy or radiotherapy. Nonetheless, men treated for localized prostate cancer commonly had declines in all functional domains during 15 years of follow-up. (Funded by the National Cancer Institute.)

▶ This is an interesting article that suggests that quality of life or functional outcomes at 15 years are very similar between these 2 modalities of treatment for localized carcinoma of the prostate. However, at 2 and 5 years, there were substantial differences in urinary incontinence and erectile dysfunction in favor of radiotherapy. From a surgical perspective, this is somewhat sobering. However, the groups studied herein are not equivalent, and, thus, the findings can be interpreted in a variety of ways. Because this is a retrospective study, the groups are not matched, and considerable selection bias may exist in the selection of the patients undergoing each of the therapies. This is suggested by the somewhat older and more sick (more comorbidities) individuals undergoing radiation therapy compared with surgery. Additionally, a substantial number of the individuals treated in both groups had low-grade disease (total Gleason score 4 or less), who today might be relegated to less-invasive treatment.

E. S. Rovner, MD

11 Voiding Dysfunction/ Enuresis

Urodynamic Studies in Adults: AUA/SUFU Guideline
Winters JC, Dmochowski RR, Goldman HB, et al (American Urological Association Education and Res, Inc, Linthicum, MD; Female Pelvic Medicine and Urogenital Reconstruction, Las Vegas, NV)
J Urol 188:2464-2472, 2012

Purpose.—The authors of this guideline reviewed the literature regarding use of urodynamic testing in common lower urinary tract symptoms. The findings are intended to assist clinicians in the appropriate selection of urodynamic tests, following an evaluation and symptom characterization.

Materials and Methods.—A systematic review of the literature using the MEDLINE® and EMBASE databases (searched from 1/1/90 to 3/10/11) was conducted to identify peer-reviewed publications relevant to using urodynamic tests for diagnosis, determining prognosis, guiding clinical management decisions and improving patient outcomes in patients with various urologic conditions. The review yielded an evidence base of 393 studies after application of inclusion/exclusion criteria. These publications were used to create the evidence basis for characterizing the statements presented in the guideline as Standards, Recommendations or Options. When sufficient evidence existed, the body of evidence for a particular treatment was assigned a strength rating of A (high), B (moderate) or C (low). In the absence of sufficient evidence, additional information is provided as Clinical Principles and Expert Opinion.

Results.—The evidence-based guideline statements are provided for diagnosis and overall management of common LUTS conditions.

Conclusions.—The Panel recognizes that each patient presenting with LUTS is unique. This Guideline is intended to serve as a tool facilitating the most effective utilization of urodynamic testing as part of a comprehensive evaluation of patients presenting with LUTS.

▶ This guideline document is the result of an intensive evidenced-based review of the urodynamics literature; however, many of the recommendations are based on expert opinion. More than 390 studies were reviewed to yield this document, and it is noteworthy that there were very few Level 1 randomized trials on which recommendations could be based. Nevertheless, some useful guidance was provided.

- Urethral function should be assessed if it will alter management (ie, leak point pressure or urethral closure pressure).
- Elevated postvoid residual (PVR) suggests detrusor underactivity bladder outlet obstruction (BOO) and potentially an increased risk for postoperative voiding difficulty.
- Repeat stress testing with the urethral catheter removed is important in those suspected of stress urinary incontinence who do not initially demonstrate such findings on initial testing.
- Urodynamic studies (UDS) may be used to evaluate for BOO in patients with urge urinary incontinence after bladder outlet procedures.
- Absence of detrusor overactivity on a single UDS study does not exclude it as a cause of patients' symptoms.
- PVR should be assessed in those with neurologic conditions and systemic conditions, including AIDS, chronic alcohol use, diabetes, myelomeningocele, and radical pelvic surgery.
- A cystometrogram (CMG) is recommended at the time of initial consult for neurogenic patients, or after spinal shock phase in those with spinal cord injury, even in the absence of symptoms. In such patients, CMG may be useful in assessing the risk of renal complications.
- Video UDS is useful in evaluating the lower urinary tract in those with neurologic disease.
- In men with lower urinary tract symptoms, obstruction on a pressure-flow study predicts better outcomes from surgery than a diagnosis of no obstruction.

E. S. Rovner, MD

Patterns and Predictors of Urodynamics Use in the United States
Reynolds WS, Penson and the Urologic Diseases in America Project (Vanderbilt Univ Med Ctr, Nashville, TN; et al)
J Urol 189:1791-1796, 2013

Purpose.—Due to the paucity of data on urodynamics on the national level, we assessed the use of urodynamics in a large sample of individuals in the United States and identified predictors of increased complexity of urodynamic procedures.

Materials and Methods.—Using administrative health care claims for adults enrolled in private insurance plans in the United States from 2002 to 2007, we identified those who underwent cystometrogram and abstracted relevant demographic and clinical data. We used logistic regression to identify predictors of higher urodynamic complexity over basic cystometrogram, specifically cystometrogram plus pressure flow study and videourodynamics.

Results.—We identified 16,574 urodynamic studies, of which 23% were cystometrograms, 71% were cystometrograms plus pressure flow studies and 6% were videourodynamics. Stress incontinence was the most common clinical condition for all studies (33.7%), cystometrogram (30.8%), cystometrogram plus pressure flow study (35.4%) and videourodynamics (24.4%). Urologists performed 59.8% of all urodynamics and gynecologists performed 35.5%. Providers with 14 or more urodynamic studies during the study period performed 75% of all urodynamics and were more likely to perform cystometrogram plus pressure flow study and videourodynamics. On regression analysis the most consistent predictors of cystometrogram plus pressure flow study and/or videourodynamics over cystometrogram were specialty (urologist) and the number of urodynamic tests performed by the provider.

Conclusions.—Most urodynamics in this series consisted of cystometrogram plus pressure flow study with stress incontinence the most common diagnosis. However, regardless of diagnosis, urologists and providers who performed more urodynamics were more likely to perform pressure flow study and/or videourodynamics in addition to cystometrogram. Further research is needed to determine whether these differences reflect gaps in the consistency or appropriateness of using urodynamics.

▶ I was surprised to see that most urodynamics studies (83%) were performed in women. However, it is important to note that the analysis was conducted on a dataset of younger, employed individuals (mean age 53.0 years). I suspect that a similar analysis using Medicare data would show a significantly greater proportion of men who undergo urodynamics because of the presence of voiding symptoms, benign prostatic hyperplasia, and urinary retention in older men. The authors discuss controversies related to the role of urodynamics in female stress incontinence and pelvic prolapse. It is important to reinforce that pressure-flow studies remain the reference standard for the diagnosis of bladder outlet obstruction in men and that identification of the presence of urodynamic bladder outlet obstruction predicts a better outcome from surgery than a finding of no obstruction.[1]

.J. Quentin Clemens, MD

Reference

1. Winters JC, Dmochowski RR, Goldman HB, et al; *Adult Urodynamics: AUA/SUFU Guideline.* Linthicum, MD: American Urological Association Education and Research 2012.

Diagnosis and Treatment of Overactive Bladder (Non-Neurogenic) in Adults: AUA/SUFU Guideline

Gormley EA, Lightner DJ, Burgio KL, et al (American Urological Association Education and Res, Inc, Linthicum, MD; Society of Urodynamics, Female Pelvic Medicine and Urogenital Reconstruction, Las Vegas, NV)
J Urol 188:2455-2463, 2012

Purpose.—The purpose of this guideline is to provide a clinical framework for the diagnosis and treatment of non-neurogenic overactive bladder (OAB).

Materials and Methods.—The primary source of evidence for this guideline is the systematic review and data extraction conducted as part of the Agency for Healthcare Research and Quality (AHRQ) Evidence Report/Technology Assessment Number 187 titled *Treatment of Overactive Bladder in Women* (2009). That report searched PubMed, MEDLINE®, EMBASE and CINAHL for English-language studies published from January 1966 to October 2008. The AUA conducted additional literature searches to capture treatments not covered in detail by the AHRQ report and relevant articles published between October 2008 and December 2011. The review yielded an evidence base of 151 treatment articles after application of inclusion/exclusion criteria. When sufficient evidence existed, the body of evidence for a particular treatment was assigned a strength rating of A (high), B (moderate) or C (low). Additional treatment information is provided as Clinical Principles and Expert Opinions when insufficient evidence existed.

Results.—The evidence-based guideline statements are provided for diagnosis and overall management of the adult with OAB symptoms as well as for various treatments. The panel identified first through third line treatments as well as non-FDA approved, rarely applicable and treatments that should not be offered.

Conclusions.—The evidence-based statements are provided for diagnosis and overall management of OAB, as well as for the various treatments. Diagnosis and treatment methodologies can be expected to change as the evidence base grows and as new treatment strategies become obtainable.

▶ The treatment of overactive bladder (OAB) continues to evolve. Underscoring this is that this evidence-based review provided contemporary and timely recommendations regarding the initial evaluation and treatment of OAB; however, since its publication in November 2012, 2 additional treatments have already been approved in the US (OnabotulinumtoxinA and Mirabegron) and more are in development. To the credit of the authors, both the evaluation and treatment guidelines are delineated in a clear, sequential fashion that is easy to understand and are consistent with most current treatment paradigms.

E. S. Rovner, MD

Efficacy and Tolerability of Mirabegron, a β₃-Adrenoceptor Agonist, in Patients with Overactive Bladder: Results from a Randomised European–Australian Phase 3 Trial

Khullar V, Amarenco G, Angulo JC, et al (Imperial College, London, UK; Hôpital Tenon, Paris, France; Hospital Universitario de Getafe, Madrid, Spain; et al)

Eur Urol 63:283-295, 2013

Background.—Mirabegron, a β₃-adrenoceptor agonist, has been developed for the treatment of overactive bladder (OAB).

Objective.—To assess the efficacy and tolerability of mirabegron versus placebo.

Design, Setting, and Participants.—Multicenter randomised double-blind, parallel-group placebo- and tolterodine-controlled phase 3 trial conducted in 27 countries in Europe and Australia in patients ≥18 yr of age with symptoms of OAB for ≥3 mo.

Intervention.—After a 2-wk single-blind placebo run-in period, patients were randomised to receive placebo, mirabegron 50 mg, mirabegron 100 mg, or tolterodine extended release 4 mg orally once daily for 12 wk.

Outcome Measurements and Statistical Analysis.—Patients completed a micturition diary and quality-of-life (QoL) assessments. Co—primary efficacy end points were change from baseline to final visit in the mean number of incontinence episodes and micturitions per 24 h. The primary comparison was between mirabegron and placebo with a secondary comparison between tolterodine and placebo. Safety parameters included adverse events (AEs), laboratory assessments, vital signs, electrocardiograms, and postvoid residual volume.

Results and Limitations.—A total of 1978 patients were randomised and received the study drug. Mirabegron 50-mg and 100-mg groups demonstrated statistically significant improvements (adjusted mean change from baseline [95% confidence intervals]) at the final visit in the number of incontinence episodes per 24 h (−1.57 [−1.79 to −1.35] and −1.46 [−1.68 to −1.23], respectively, vs placebo −1.17 [−1.39 to −0.95]) and number of micturitions per 24 h (−1.93 [−2.15 to −1.72] and −1.77 [−1.99 to −1.56], respectively, vs placebo −1.34 [−1.55 to −1.12]; $p < 0.05$ for all comparisons). Statistically significant improvements were also observed in other key efficacy end points and QoL outcomes. The incidence of treatment-emergent AEs was similar across treatment groups. The main limitation of this study was the short (12-wk) duration of treatment.

Conclusions.—Mirabegron represents a new class of treatment for OAB with proven efficacy and good tolerability.

Trial Identification.—This study is registered at ClinicalTrials.gov, identifier NCT00689104.

▶ Mirabegron represents the first in a new class of agents for the treatment of overactive bladder. These efficacy data are interesting, but the most remarkable finding was the absence of the side effects seen with antimuscarinic agents. The incidence of xerostomia and constipation were quite low. This is to be expected because mirabegron is not an antimuscarinic agent and therefore would not be expected to have such side effects. The cardiovascular safety profile was satisfactory in this study. Whether beta-3 agonists will be more efficacious or safer as compared with antimuscarinics remains to be seen.

E. S. Rovner, MD

Long-term outcome of the use of intravesical botulinum toxin for the treatment of overactive bladder (OAB)

Mohee A, Khan A, Harris N, et al (St James Univ Hosp, Leeds, UK)
BJU Int 111:106-113, 2013

Objectives.—• To assess the long-term compliance with repeated injections of intravesical botulinum toxin (BT) in a 'real-life' mixed population of patients with idiopathic detrusor overactivity and neurogenic detrusor overactivity.

• To identify the reasons why patients discontinued BT therapy and to explore the outcomes of those patients who did discontinue treatment.

Patients and Methods.—• Retrospective evaluation of the case notes of a series of patients who had received intravesical BT treatment at a large UK teaching hospital.

• No antibiotic prophylaxis was given for the procedure.

Results.—• Over a period of 7 years, 268 patients were initiated on intravesical BT treatment for overactive bladder (OAB) at our institution, with 137 followed up for ≥36 months, with 80 patients having ≥60 months follow-up after their first injection.

• Almost two-thirds of patients (61.3%) had discontinued intravesical BT therapy at 36 months, with a 63.8% discontinuation rate at 60 months.

• The main reasons for discontinuation were tolerability issues, mainly urinary tract infections and the need for clean intermittent self-catheterisation. Primary and secondary losses of efficacy were of secondary importance.

• Most of the patients that discontinued have remained under urology care and now receive alternative methods of treatment.

Conclusions.—• Intravesical BT therapy is an effective short-term treatment for OAB.

• With time, two-thirds of patients discontinued treatment usually because of the tolerability issues associated with treatment.

▶ The long-term effectiveness of botulinum toxin therapy for the treatment of idiopathic overactive bladder is not known. Persistence with treatment is dependent on numerous factors, including efficacy of the treatment in reducing symptoms, side effects, availability of other treatment options, and financial impact to the patient. This study suggests that persistence with botulinum toxin therapy at 5 years is relatively low, with only 36% of patients continuing with the treatments at that time point. Major reasons for discontinuation were related to UTIs and urinary retention. However, most patients were treated with a 200-U dose of onabotulinumtoxinA, and subsequent studies have indicated that a dose of 100 U is associated with similar efficacy but a lower rate of urinary retention. Therefore, one would expect greater persistence with therapy if a 100-U dose had been utilized.

The injections were initially performed under general anesthesia, utilizing 30 injection sites. Over time, the technique was transitioned to 10 injection sites, performed under local anesthesia. This exactly mirrors my practice, in which virtually all botulinum toxin injections are now performed in the office, using 10 mL of botulinum solution delivered in 1 mL increments, regardless of the dose (100, 200, or 300 U).

J. Quentin Clemens, MD

Increased Risk of Large Post-Void Residual Urine and Decreased Long-Term Success Rate After Intravesical OnabotulinumtoxinA Injection for Refractory Idiopathic Detrusor Overactivity
Liao C-H, Kuo H-C (Fu-Jen Catholic Univ, Hualien, Taiwan, Republic of China; Tzu Chi Univ, Hualien, Taiwan, Republic of China)
J Urol 189:1804-1810, 2013

Purpose.—Intravesical injection of onabotulinumtoxinA is effective for idiopathic detrusor overactivity refractory to antimuscarinics. However, safety is a major concern, especially in elderly individuals. We investigated the efficacy and safety of intravesical onabotulinumtoxinA injection for refractory idiopathic detrusor overactivity in the frail elderly population.

Materials and Methods.—A total of 166 patients with urodynamic idiopathic detrusor overactivity refractory to previous antimuscarinics for more than 3 months received 1 intravesical 100 U onabotulinumtoxinA injection from 2004 to 2009. Frail elderly was defined as age greater than 65 years and 3 or more of certain criteria, including unintentional weight loss, self-reported exhaustion, weakness, slow walking speed and/or low physical activity. Treatment results were assessed by the Patient Perception of Bladder Condition, voiding diary, urodynamic parameters and Kaplan-Meier estimates of survival plots.

Results.—We evaluated 61 frail elderly patients, 63 who were elderly without frailty and 42 younger than 65 years. Large post-void residual urine volume (greater than 150 ml) after onabotulinumtoxinA injection was significantly higher in the frail elderly group than in the other groups (60.7% vs 39.7% and 35.7%, respectively, $p = 0.018$). Urinary retention developed in 7 frail elderly patients (11.5%), 4 (6.3%) who were elderly without frailty and 1 younger patient (2.4%) ($p = 0.203$). Recovery duration was significantly longer in frail elderly patients. The cumulative success rate was significantly lower in the frail elderly group than in the other 2 groups ($p = 0.009$).

Conclusions.—Although safety and efficacy were similar between elderly patients without frailty and younger patients, an increased risk of large post-void residual urine volume and a lower long-term success rate in frail elderly patients were noted after intravesical onabotulinumtoxinA injection for refractory idiopathic detrusor overactivity.

▶ The title of this article does not really convey what was done. The authors identified a cohort of frail elderly who had undergone onabotulinumtoxinA injections (100 U dose) for idiopathic detrusor overactivity, and compared their results with a cohort of nonfrail elderly and a cohort of younger patients. Approximately half of these subjects were men. The mean age of the elderly patients was 75 years, and the mean age of the younger patients was 45 years. The methods used to identify frailty seem reasonable, but it appears that this was done via retrospective chart review, and these methods are apparently not validated. Nevertheless, the results seem to make sense. Success rates at 3 and 6 months were similar across all 3 groups but were lower in the frail elderly group at 12 months. More importantly, the frail elderly showed greater postvoid residual volumes and a higher rate of symptomatic urinary retention. If urinary retention did develop, the frail elderly took a longer time to resume voiding. The main message appears to be that onabotulinumtoxinA is effective in the frail elderly but is associated with greater side effects. Although this may seem intuitive, this is the first study to clearly demonstrate these findings.

J. Quentin Clemens, MD

Sacral Neuromodulation with an Implantable Pulse Generator in Children With Lower Urinary Tract Symptoms: 15-Year Experience
Groen L-A, Hoebeke P, Loret N, et al (Ghent Univ Hosp, Belgium)
J Urol 188:1313-1317, 2012

Purpose.—Sacral nerve modulation with an implantable pulse generator is not an established treatment in children. This therapy has been described for dysfunctional elimination syndrome and neurogenic bladder. We report 2 new indications for this approach in children, ie bladder overactivity and Fowler syndrome. The aim of this study was to improve the results of future treatment for sacral neuromodulation in children by describing factors favorable for good outcomes with this method.

Materials and Methods.—A total of 18 children 9 to 17 years old were studied. Mean ± SD followup was 28.8 ± 43.8 months. Of the patients 16 underwent S3 sacral neuromodulation and 7 underwent pudendal stimulation (5 as a revision, 2 from the beginning).

Results.—Initial full response was achieved in 9 of 18 patients (50%) and partial response in 5 (28%). In patients presenting with incontinence mean ± SD number of incontinence episodes weekly improved significantly from 23.2 ± 12.4 to 1.3 ± 2.63 (p <0.05). In patients requiring clean intermittent catheterization there was a significant decrease in mean ± SD daily frequency of catheterization from 5.2 ± 1.6 to 2.0 ± 1.9 (p <0.05). At the end of the study 6 of 15 patients (40%) had a full response and 5 (33%) had a partial response, while 4 implantable pulse generator devices (27%) were explanted because of failure.

Conclusions.—Sacral neuromodulation is feasible in the pediatric population, with good short-term (78% full or partial response) and satisfactory long-term results (73%). Sacral neuromodulation can offer good results for overactive bladder, dysfunctional elimination syndrome and Fowler syndrome. Pudendal nerve stimulation is a feasible salvage treatment that can be useful in cases when S3 implantation is impossible or unsuccessful.

▶ Sacral nerve modulation (IPG) is approved in adults with voiding symptomatology refractory to pelvic muscle rehabilitation and anticholinergics. It is not approved in neurogenic bladder dysfunction. It is unclear in my mind that abnormal nerves can be modulated. The authors show that IPG does have some efficacy (60%) in both underactive and overactive bladders. There was a full response in only 6 of 18 patients. The IPG was used in 3 patients with a neurogenic bladder, and there was no response. Urodynamics were not performed before and after test stimulation. These data would be especially useful in children with a neurogenic bladder. The procedure is expensive and the reoperation rate is high, but IPG may have some utility in children with refractory nonneurogenic voiding dysfunction.

D. E. Coplen, MD

The prevalence and natural history of urinary symptoms among recreational ketamine users

Winstock AR, Mitcheson L, Gillatt DA, et al (South London and Maudsley NHS Foundation Trust St George's Hosp Med School, London, UK; Southmead Hosp, Bristol, UK)

BJU Int 110:1762-1766, 2012

Objective.—• To investigate the prevalence and natural history of urinary symptoms in a cohort of recreational ketamine users.

Patients and Methods.—• A purposeful sampling technique was used.

• Between November 2009 and January 2010 participants were invited to undertake an on-line questionnaire promoted by a national dance music magazine and website.

• Data regarding demographics and illicit drug-use were collected.

• Among respondents reporting recent ketamine use, additional information detailing their ketamine use, experience of urinary symptoms and use of related healthcare services was obtained.

Results.—• In all, 3806 surveys were completed, of which 1285 (33.8%) participants reported ketamine use within the last year.

• Of the ketamine users, 17% were found to be dependent on the drug; 26.6% (340) of recent ketamine users reported experiencing urinary symptoms.

• Urinary symptoms were significantly related to both dose of ketamine used and frequency of ketamine use.

• Of 251 users reporting their experience of symptoms over time in relationship to their use of ketamine, 51% reported improvement in urinary symptoms upon cessation of use with only eight (3.8%) reporting deterioration after stopping use.

Conclusions.—• Urinary tract symptoms are reported in over a quarter of regular ketamine users.

• A dose and frequency response relationship has been shown between ketamine use and urinary symptoms.

• Both users and primary-care providers need to be educated about urinary symptoms that may arise in ketamine users. A multi-disciplinary approach promoting harm reduction, cessation and early referral is needed to manage individuals with ketamine-associated urinary tract symptoms to avoid progression to severe and irreversible urological pathologies.

What's known on the subject? and What does the study add?

Case series have described lower urinary tract symptoms associated with ketamine use including severe pain, frequency, haematuria and dysuria. Little is known regarding the frequency of symptoms, relationship of symptoms with dose and frequency of use and natural history of symptoms once the ketamine user has stopped.

This study describes the prevalence of ketamine use in a population of recreational drug users in a dance music setting. It shows a dose—frequency relationship with ketamine use. It shows that urinary symptoms associated with recreational ketamine use may lead to a considerable demand on health resources in the primary-, secondary- and emergency-care settings. It shows that symptoms may improve once ketamine use is decreased.

Study Type.—Symptom prevalence (prospective cohort).
Level of Evidence.—1b.

▶ Recreational use of ketamine is apparently commonplace in certain Asian countries, and its use appears to be increasing in the United Kingdom as well. The use of ketamine has been associated with the development of lower urinary tract symptoms such as frequency, urgency, dysuria, and hematuria. The symptoms can progress to end-stage bladder dysfunction with hydronephrosis and renal failure. The pathophysiology of ketamine-induced bladder dysfunction is not clear at this time. This survey of 1285 ketamine users in the United Kingdom indicates that approximately 25% of users will experience urinary symptoms and that the presence of these symptoms is dose related. Fortunately, the symptoms appear to resolve in most users after cessation of ketamine use. Recreational ketamine use in the United States appears to be low at this time, although it almost certainly does exist. In younger individuals with idiopathic lower urinary tract symptoms, it seems prudent to inquire about ketamine use.

J. Quentin Clemens, MD

Experience with Glycerin for Antegrade Continence Enema in Patients with Neurogenic Bowel
Chu DI, Balsara ZR, Routh JC, et al (Duke Univ Med Ctr, Durham, NC)
J Urol 189:690-693, 2013

Purpose.—Malone antegrade continence enemas are used in the management of neurogenic bowel to attain fecal continence. Several different irrigation solutions have been described but glycerin, an osmotic laxative that promotes peristalsis, has rarely been mentioned or studied. We assessed clinical outcomes in our patients with a Malone antegrade continence enema using glycerin based irrigation.

Materials and Methods.—We retrospectively reviewed patients with neurogenic bowel who underwent a Malone antegrade continence enema procedure between 1997 and 2011. Glycerin diluted with tap water followed by a tap water flush is our preferred irrigation protocol. Bowel regimen outcomes examined included fecal continence, emptying time, leakage from stoma, enema volume, frequency and independence.

Results.—Of the 23 patients with followup greater than 6 months 19 used glycerin based irrigation. Average age at surgery was 8.8 years. Patients using glycerin instilled a median of 30 ml (mean 29) glycerin and 50 ml (131) tap water. Fecal continence rate was 95% and stoma leakage rate was 16%, and only 16% of patients required daily irrigation.

Conclusions.—Glycerin is a viable and effective alternative irrigant for antegrade enemas of neurogenic bowel, with an excellent fecal continence rate. The volume of irrigant needed is typically less than 90 ml, which is much less than in published reports using tap water alone.

▶ Management of chronic constipation and fecal incontinence in patients with neurogenic bowel dysfunction can be challenging. A small percentage of patients have continence with stool softeners and timed defecation. Retrograde enemas are typically ineffective unless used with a cone or plug that occludes the anus to prevent efflux until the entire volume is instilled. Even if a retrograde enema is efficacious, self-administration is difficult in patients with poor mobility. Antegrade enema via a catheterizable colonic stoma or button was first described by Malone in 1990. Saline, tap water, polyethylene glycol, and mineral oil have been used as irrigants. Continence with this technique is excellent. However, in patients with a very redundant colon, the irrigation volumes are often very large (1 L), and the evacuation time often exceeds an hour.

The authors describe the addition of glycerin to the irrigant. Glycerin has been well studied in suppositories and retrograde enemas and is safe with minimal cramping as a side effect. This acts as an osmotic laxative that promotes peristalsis. The patients were able to decrease the instilled volumes without a change in bowel continence when compared with tap water alone. However, the mean evacuation time after enema was still 45 minutes. This is a small sample size, and there is no direct comparison with other irrigants. This approach warrants further evaluation.

D. E. Coplen, MD

Bladder and bowel dysfunction and the resolution of urinary incontinence with successful management of bowel symptoms in children

Borch L, Hagstroem S, Bower WF, et al (Aarhus Univ Hosp, Skejby, Denmark; Aarhus Univ Hosp, Aalborg, Denmark)
Acta Paediatr 102:e215-e220, 2013

Aim.—To investigate the effect of treating defecation problems on urinary incontinence in children suffering from combined urinary bladder and bowel dysfunction (BBD).

Methods.—We established a clinical database from medical records of all children referred to the urinary incontinence and gastroenterology outpatient clinics with BBD. The following variables were extracted: symptoms of constipation, faecal incontinence, urinary incontinence, age at onset of symptoms, treatment, including duration and response. All children went through the same treatment protocol. Faecal disorders were treated primarily and once relieved, the daytime incontinence was managed and followed by intervention for nocturnal enuresis.

Results.—In total, 73 children were included in the study. The treatment regimen resulted in resolution of the defecation disorder in 96% of the patients. Of the children with daytime urinary incontinence, 68% had at least a 50% reduction in number of daytime incontinence episodes by successful relief of bowel dysfunction and 27% became completely continent during daytime. Only 17% of the children suffering from enuresis had a significant reduction in number of wet nights after relief of their faecal problem.

Conclusion.—The empirical treatment approach of managing bowel symptoms before intervening for bladder dysfunction in children with BBD is found to be appropriate.

▶ The impact of constipation on bladder function should not be underestimated. Unless there is fecal soiling or incontinence, parents are often completely unaware of the character and frequency of their children's bowel movements. Consequently, they are often reluctant to accept that their child has bowel issues and are unwilling to initiate any therapy for them. The Bristol scale is a visual representation of different stool types with pebbly and voluminous hard stool being representative of constipation. The Rome III criteria are the accepted standard for defining constipation (≤ 2 bowel movements per week, fecal incontinence, painful or hard, large diameter plugging the toilet, retentive posturing).

In this study, most children (n = 58) were referred for treatment of urinary incontinence. Referring physicians had concerns regarding constipation or gastrointestinal issues in only 15. Eighty-four percent of children referred for evaluation of urinary incontinence had at least 2 Rome III criteria for constipation. All children were treated to achieve normal bowel habits (timed sitting and laxatives) before any discussion regarding treatment for urinary incontinence (eg, voiding diaries, timed voiding). Children with refractory bowel symptoms were excluded from the analysis. There was marked improvement in urinary symptoms when fecal elimination improved. The exact reason is not clear. Some of this may be purely mechanical. In many cases, however, the bowel symptoms are related to neuromuscular dysfunction, and improved coordination eventually results in improved urinary continence. Because constipation plays such an important role, there is rarely a role for anticholinergics, which typically exacerbate constipation. Empirical first-line treatment is appropriate because most children with urinary symptoms also have incontinence.

D. E. Coplen, MD

12 Sexual Function

Sexual Dysfunction among Male Veterans Returning from Iraq and Afghanistan: Prevalence and Correlates
Hosain GMM, Latini DM, Kauth M, et al (Houston VA HSR&D Ctr of Excellence, TX; et al)
J Sex Med 10:516-523, 2013

Introduction.—Sexual dysfunction (SD) is not well described in the Iraq/ Afghanistan veteran population despite high prevalence of multiple risk factors for this issue.

Aim.—To estimate the prevalence and examine the association of various sociodemographic, mental health, comorbid conditions and life style factors with sexual dysfunction in Iraq/Afghanistan veterans.

Methods.—This exploratory cross-sectional study was conducted using data from the VA administrative database. A total of 4,755 Iraq/Afghanistan veterans were identified who sought treatment from the Michael E. DeBakey Veterans Affairs Medical Center inpatient and outpatient clinic between September 2007 and August 2009.

Main Outcome Measures.—Sexual dysfunction was determined by ICD9-CM codes related to sexual health issues and/or by specific medications, primarily phosphodiesterase-5 inhibitors (PDE5i), prescribed for erectile dysfunction.

Results.—The overall prevalence of sexual dysfunction was 5.5% (N = 265). By age category, it was 3.6% (N = 145) for Iraq/Afghanistan veterans aged 18–40 years and 15.7% (N = 120) for Iraq/Afghanistan veterans aged >40 years, respectively. A multivariate logistic-regression model revealed that annual income, marital status, post-traumatic stress disorder, and hypertension were significant risk factors of SD (all $P < 0.05$) among younger Iraq/Afghanistan veterans, whereas among the older Iraq/ Afghanistan veterans, being African American and having PTSD and hypertension were significant risk factors of SD (all $P < 0.05$). There was marked discrepancy between documented erectile dysfunction and prescription of a PDE5i.

Conclusions.—These data demonstrate that a significant proportion of Iraq/Afghanistan veterans have SD and that the risk factors differ between younger and older veterans. Our findings also suggest that SD is likely under-coded. To better identify the scope of the problem, systematic screening for sexual dysfunction may be appropriate perhaps as part of an initial post-deployment health evaluation.

▶ The winding down of US military intervention overseas is a welcome development for many important reasons. The long-standing obligation of our medical community to provide for our wounded soldiers is more challenging than ever secondary to our improved ability to save lives in combat situations; soldiers who would have died of injuries in the past now survive and are in need of intensive rehabilitation and medical attention.

Provision of sexual medicine services and promotion of sexual wellness is an important part of our mandate to care for our veterans. This important study examines sexual dysfunction (based on 10 ICD9 codes relating to sexual dysfunction) in this young, generally healthy, and potentially reproductively minded cohort of individuals. Posttraumatic stress disorder emerged as an important predictive factor for sexual dysfunction in both young (18–40 years) and older (> 40 years) groups. In addition, the standard risk factors for sexual dysfunction (eg, relationship status, vascular disease, depression) remained important risk factors for sexual dysfunction as well.

A. W. Shindel, MD

Bother and distress associated with Peyronie's disease: validation of the Peyronie's Disease Questionnaire (PDQ)

Hellstrom WJG, Feldman R, Rosen RC, et al (Tulane Univ Health Sciences Ctr, New Orleans, LA; Connecticut Clinical Res Ctr, Middlebury; New England Res Insts, Inc, Watertown, MA; et al)

J Urol 2013 [Epub ahead of print]

Purpose.—To validate the Peyronie's Disease Questionnaire (PDQ), a 15-question self-reported survey, measuring the impact and severity of Peyronie's disease (PD) symptoms in 3 domains: 1) Psychological and Physical Symptoms, 2) Penile Pain, and 3) Symptom Bother.

Materials and Methods.—Baseline data from two phase 3 clinical trials of collagenase clostridium histolyticum for the treatment of PD-associated penile curvature and bother were used (N = 334; N = 345). Collected data included PDQ domain scores (full PDQ available at http://www.auxilium. com/PDQ), International Index of Erectile Function (IIEF) scores, objective measures of penile curvature, and subject-reported PD symptom severity. The Psychometric analyses included confirmatory factor analyses (CFAs), inter-item reliability, and tests of convergent and discriminant validity, all related to the overall construct validity of the scale.

Results.—CFAs supported the conceptual framework of the PDQ with 3 confirmed sub-domains. Good consistency (i.e., internal reliability) of each scale was demonstrated (all Cronbach's alphas >0.70). Convergent and discriminant validity were shown in the pattern of associations between PDQ domains and other measures of PD. PDQ domain scores significantly differed between patients with or without ED and between patients with or without PD-related symptom distress, further supporting the construct validity of the PDQ.

Conclusions.—This study confirms the conceptual framework, factor structure, and convergent and discriminant validity of the PDQ Psychological and Physical Symptoms, Penile Pain, and Symptom Bother domains. Used in conjunction with objective penile curvature measurements, the PDQ can serve as a valuable diagnostic tool or outcome measure for assessing treatment-related improvements in PD symptoms.

▶ We have an ever-expanding cornucopia of survey tools to assess sexuality-related distress and erectile dysfunction (ED) in particular. There is an emerging selection of tools to assess premature ejaculation (PE). Unfortunately, validated patient-reported metrics for Peyronie disease (PD) are (or were) lacking. This is an important absence, as the metrics currently used for PE and ED will not accurately and precisely capture the experiences of men with PD.

This publication represents validation of the first tool for precise assessment of the impact of PD in men. This is an important step forward, primarily for research and assessment of results but also potentially for the clinical assessment of patients and their response to individual therapies. Subclassification of symptoms into psychological/physical symptoms, penile pain, and symptom bother permits assessment of the multidimensional nature of the condition.

The complex modeling and statistical analysis that go into development of these criteria make for very dense reading; nevertheless, the results of the in-depth analysis were supportive of this instrument's usefulness in the setting of PD.

A. W. Shindel, MD

Psychological Impact of Peyronie's Disease: A Review
Nelson CJ, Mulhall JP (Memorial Sloan-Kettering Cancer Ctr, NY)
J Sex Med 10:653-660, 2013

Introduction.—Peyronie's disease (PD) is characterized by an accumulation of scar tissue in the tunica albuginea of the penis that causes curvature and deformity. PD can result in psychological distress, depression, or anxiety, which often goes untreated.

Aims.—To review the current literature on the psychological impact of PD, educate healthcare providers about the psychological components of the disease, and propose interventions that address the psychological and sexual challenges patients and their partners may encounter.

Methods.—We performed a MEDLINE search, limited to English, using the terms "Peyronie's disease" AND "psychological" OR "psychosocial," and select references were included for review.

Main Outcome Measure.—Critical review of the currently available English language literature.

Results.—PD and its associated deformity often impairs sexual relations and frequently leads to psychological and psychosocial sequelae for affected individuals. Many men experience depression, low self-esteem, and emotional distress; these problems markedly diminish the quality of life for affected individuals. The literature suggests that as many as 81% of men report "emotional difficulties," 48% report clinically meaningful depression (26% moderate; 21% severe), and 54% report relationship problems due to PD. The challenges imposed by PD include alterations in sexual relationships, restrictions on intimacy, social isolation, and stigmatization, all of which are linked and reinforce each other. Physicians may be unaware of the psychological sequelae suffered by patients and their partners.

Conclusions.—Improved awareness and education about the psychological consequences and treatment options for PD are necessary among healthcare providers. To best help patients and optimize outcomes, a team-based approach is needed that includes psychosocial assessment and appropriate resource referrals for the patient and his sexual partner.

▶ Most urologists don't like dealing with Peyronie disease. It's not surprising; we don't really understand what causes it, we don't have a universally agreed upon way to treat it, and the patients often present with very marked distress.

This article underscores why it is important that we continue to stay invested in the treatment (and as importantly, research) of Peyronie's. The psychological impacts of this disease are devastating, in part because most men (and many doctors) don't know that a condition like this exists. Erectile dysfunction and premature ejaculation are in the common parlance, but Peyronie disease is a term unfamiliar to most of the public.

The results are highlighted here; more than half of men report relationship problems from the condition. More than 4 in 5 have emotional difficulty with it. This underscores the importance of involving psychological support in the care of the patient. This is obviously somewhat beyond the expertise of most urologists, but I would recommend that a mechanism for referral to an appropriate sex therapist or counselor might be useful in some of these cases. The Association of Peyronie Disease Advocates is another valuable resource; this website is patient-run and provides a community for discussion and support. More info can be obtained at www.peyroniesassocation.org.

A. W. Shindel, MD

Listening to Placebo in Clinical Trials for Female Sexual Dysfunction
Bradford A (Univ of Texas MD Anderson Cancer Ctr, Houston)
J Sex Med 10:451-459, 2013

Introduction.—Placebo responses are substantial in many clinical trials of treatments for female sexual dysfunctions (FSDs). Recent studies from other fields suggest a need to reconceptualize placebo response and to design future trials accordingly.

Aim.—The aims of this review are to (i) summarize current conceptualizations of placebo response in the literature; (ii) identify potential mechanisms of placebo response that are relevant to the study of FSD; and (iii) provide recommendations for incorporating this knowledge into design of future trials.

Methods.—Narrative review of literature relevant to the topic of placebo response and FSD.

Main Outcome Measures.—Possible predictors and mechanisms of placebo response in women with FSD are described based on the synthesis of empirical findings in studies of placebo.

Results.—Placebo response is a complex phenomenon that represents cognitive, behavioral, motivational, and possibly relational mediating factors. Instructions given to trial participants, behavioral changes required to participate in a trial, changes in partner behavior, and interactions with study staff may influence participants' expectations of benefit and therefore their responses to placebo treatment. Side effects may enhance placebo response within active treatment arms. At present, it is unclear to what extent to which specific factors affect outcomes of clinical trials in FSD.

Conclusions.—Procedural and methodological factors are likely to contribute to placebo response in trials for FSD, though additional research is needed to clarify these effects. Study designs should be reevaluated to avoid unnecessary creation or exaggeration of placebo responses and to draw appropriate conclusions from trial results.

▶ Sexual dysfunction is of necessity a complex topic that requires very patient-centric study endpoints for research. It is difficult to reduce sexuality and sexual satisfaction to quantitative measures and objective outcome criteria. Hence, placebo effects are common, and genuine benefit from any intervention must be robust enough to overcome the high baseline rate of response in individuals who undertake any sort of therapy for their concern.

This author articulates several important concepts in placebo trials. For instance, placebo and therapeutic effects may not be additive (ie, the difference between placebo and treatment response does not necessarily represent the effect attributable to the treatment in question). Other examples include the concept that self-monitoring behavior (common in studies of sexual dysfunction) may engender change in behavior or perception regardless of treatment/placebo, or that interaction with a caring provider/researcher will induce positive change, or, most germane to sexuality research, that the partner may experience placebo by proxy and engage in behavior/attitudes that engender a positive response in the woman irrespective of her physiologic or psychological responses.

These data are not immediately applicable to clinical practice but are worth considering as the quest to identify a pharmacotherapy for women's sexual function continues.

A. W. Shindel, MD

Expression of Aquaporin Proteins in Vagina of Diabetes Mellitus Rats

Pei L, Jiang J, Jiang R, et al (Affiliated Hosp, Luzhou, China)
J Sex Med 2012 [Epub ahead of print]

Introduction.—Aquaporins (AQPs) are membrane proteins that facilitate water movement across biological membranes. Vaginal lubrication may be mediated by blood flow and other potential mechanisms related to transudation of fluid. The most common female sexual dysfunction in diabetes is inadequate vaginal lubrication.

Aim.—To investigate the expression of AQP1−3 in vaginal tissue of diabetes mellitus rats.

Methods.—Female Sprague-Dawley rats ($N = 20$) were randomly divided into group A (12-week-old nondiabetic control, $N = 5$), group B (16-week-old nondiabetes control, $N = 5$), group C (12-week-old diabetes mellitus rats, $N = 5$), and group D (16-week-old diabetes mellitus rats, $N = 5$). Vaginal fluid was measured by fluid weight absorbed by cotton swabs after pelvic nerve electrostimulation and anterior vaginal tissue was dissected for determining the expression of AQP1−3 by immunohistochemical study and Western blot.

Main Outcome Measures.—The expression of AQP1−3 was determined in the vagina of diabetes mellitus rats by Western blot.

Results.—There are no significant differences in serum estradiol concentrations of rats among these groups ($P > 0.05$). Vaginal fluid was significantly lower in group C (2.7 ± 0.67 mg) and group D (2.5 ± 1.03 mg) than in group A (5.74 ± 1.23 mg) and group B (5.5 ± 1.08 mg) ($P < 0.05$), respectively. The protein expressions of AQP1−3 were significantly lower in group C (43.40 ± 4.83, 60.60 ± 12.80, and 59.60 ± 6.95) and group D (20.81 ± 2.86, 47.80 ± 11.43, and 54.20 ± 5.26) than in group A (116.62 ± 3.21, 110.81 ± 8.044, and 108.80 ± 4.97) and group B (122.12 ± 14.54, 111.21 ± 15.07, and 106.40 ± 4.16) ($P < 0.05$), respectively.

Conclusions.—Decreased vaginal fluid in diabetes mellitus rats after electrostimulation may be partly due to estrogen-independent decreases of AQP1−3 in vaginal tissue.

▶ Vascular disease, particularly diabetes, is very clearly linked to greater risk of sexual dysfunction in men. It has been much more difficult to prove an association between vascular disease/diabetes and sexual dysfunction in women despite the opening statements of these authors' introduction section.

Some of this limitation may be due to deficiencies in our ability to accurately measure biological and psychological aspects of sexual function in women. Alternatively, one may postulate that the increase in blood flow and vasodilatation so essential to penile erection is of lesser necessity in women. Increased vaginal/clitoral engorgement and lubrication is beneficial for women's sexual enjoyment, but it may be possible for (some) women to enjoy sex without this—certainly easier than it is for most men to enjoy sex with a flaccid penis. This study is limited in that it represents just 20 rats at 2 relatively narrow time points. Whether the results can be extrapolated to humans is an important question. Still, this represents an important effort to better understand the biological underpinnings of female sexual function. More work in this direction would be most welcome.

A. W. Shindel, MD

Erectile Dysfunction Diagnosis and Treatment as a Means to Improve Medication Adherence and Optimize Comorbidity Management
Scranton RE, Goldstein I, Stecher VJ (Clinical Scientist Consulting, Framingham, MA; Alvarado Hosp, San Diego, CA; Med Affairs, Pfizer Inc, NY)
J Sex Med 2012 [Epub ahead of print]

Introduction.—Optimal pharmacologic management of diseases comorbid with erectile dysfunction (ED), such as cardiovascular disease, depression, diabetes, dyslipidemia, hypertension, and benign prostatic hyperplasia/lower urinary tract symptoms (BPH/LUTS), is dependent upon long-term treatment compliance and may be complicated by poor adherence to medication use. ED may contribute to poor adherence to medication use because poor quality erectile function may be an unwanted adverse effect of antihypertensives, antidepressants, and $5-\alpha$ reductase inhibitors for treatment of BPH/LUTS. Diminished erectile spontaneity, rigidity, and/or sustaining capability also negatively affects mood, self-esteem, and confidence, which compromise motivation to be compliant with medications that treat diseases comorbid with ED.

Aim.—Literature review was performed to explore the role of ED diagnosis and effective treatment in enhancing overall management of selected ED comorbidities, highlighting the role of medication adherence.

Methods.—Several PubMed searches were performed.

Results.—Diagnosis and successful treatment of concomitant ED may promote improved adherence and management of comorbid diseases. Concomitant ED management may improve treatment outcome, decrease healthcare costs, and possibly prevent or even improve deterioration in medical conditions comorbid with ED. Because ED is a silent marker and predictor of comorbidities, especially cardiovascular disease, earlier diagnosis of ED may provide an opportunity to prevent future cardiovascular events. In men presenting with complaints of ED, screening for, monitoring, and appropriately treating diseases that are comorbid with ED is essential. Screening for and appropriately treating ED is important for enhanced life quality and improved motivation in men with existing ED comorbidities or risk factors.

Conclusions.—Appropriate management of ED and its risk factors may have beneficial effects on diseases that are comorbid with ED, and vice versa, most likely via shared pathophysiological pathways. Clinicians may need to consider men's health overall, of which sexual health is a central component, in order to provide optimal disease management.

▶ As the biological underpinnings of sexual physiology in men have been revealed, urologists have taken an increasingly important role in the management of erectile dysfunction in men. Of course, any physician with a genuine interest in sexual wellness may take a leading role with their patients.

What does this have to do with this particular manuscript? In my opinion, this manuscript sheds light on how the urologist and/or sexual medicine physician can influence the patient's overall health by educating the patient and also primary care providers about how sexual function impacts overall health and vice versa. It's no mystery that disease states predispose patients to sexual problems; knowledge of this connection may help patients to take steps to rectify correctable causes of ill health and adhere to treatment of other comorbid conditions. Primary care physicians may find this connection particularly useful when convincing patients of the numerous benefits of healthy lifestyles (eg, diet, exercise, stress management) and/or counseling patients on sexual side effects of medications. Sincere efforts to identify patients who are noncompliant because of sexual side effects of medications may help providers find alternative solutions to medical problems.

A. W. Shindel, MD

Persistent Genital Arousal Disorder: Characterization, Etiology, and Management

Facelle TM, Sadeghi-Nejad H, Goldmeier D (UMDNJ New Jersey Med School—Surgery—Urology, Newark; Imperial College NHS Trust at St Mary's Hosp—Medicine, London, UK)
J Sex Med 2012 [Epub ahead of print]

Introduction.—Persistent genital arousal disorder (PGAD) is a potentially debilitating disorder of unwanted genital sensation and arousal that is generally spontaneous and unrelenting. Since its first description in 2001, many potential etiologies and management strategies have been suggested.

Aim.—To review the literature on PGAD, identify possible causes of the disorder, and provide approaches to the assessment and treatment of the disorder based on the authors' experience and recent literature.

Methods.—PubMed searches through July 2012 were conducted to identify articles relevant to persistent sexual arousal syndrome and PGAD.

Main Outcome Measures.—Expert opinion was based on review of the medical literature related to this subject matter.

Results.—PGAD is characterized by persistent sensations of genital arousal in the absence of sexual stimulation or emotion, which are considered unwanted and cause the patient at least moderate distress. The proposed etiologies of PGAD are plentiful and may involve a range of psychologic, pharmacologic, neurologic, and vascular causes. PGAD has been associated with other conditions including overactive bladder and restless leg syndrome. Assessment should include a through history and physical exam and tailored radiologic studies. Treatment should be aimed at reversible causes, whether physiologic or pharmacologic. All patients should be considered for cognitive therapy including mindfullness meditation and acceptance therapy.

Conclusions.—PGAD likely represents a range of conditions manifesting in unwanted genital sensations. Successful treatment requires a multidisciplinary approach and consideration of all reversible causes as well as cognitive therapy.

▶ Persistent genital arousal disorder (PGAD) has only recently been characterized but has captured the public imagination. Much like "erections lasting 4 hours or more," persistent arousal and/or recurrent orgasms have become fodder for humor and locker room mirth. This is unfortunate as all of these conditions are sources of extreme bother and social disruption—certainly no laughing matter when either of these actually happens to an individual!

PGAD is very poorly understood but has been reported in association with psychological factors (eg, history of trauma, anxiety disorder, obsessive compulsive disorder), medications (particularly antidepressants), diet (phytoestrogens), pelvic varices, central nervous system pathology, and other organic causes. It may be related to or synonymous with prior case reports of clitoral priapism. Because of poor understanding and heterogeneous potential causes, a multidisciplinary approach to assessment is advisable and should include detailed history of examination of the genitals, hormone profiles, and consideration for pelvic imaging (Doppler, magnetic resonance imaging) and/or central nervous system evaluation (electroencephalogram, magnetic resonance imaging).

A. W. Shindel, MD

Does Current Scientific and Clinical Evidence Support the Use of Phosphodiesterase Type 5 Inhibitors for the Treatment of Premature Ejaculation? A Systematic Review and Meta-analysis

Asimakopoulos AD, Miano R, Agrò EF, et al (Univ of Tor Vergata, Policlinico Casilino, Rome, Italy; Univ of Tor Vergata, Policlinico Tor Vergata, Rome, Italy)
J Sex Med 9:2404-2416, 2012

Introduction.—Premature ejaculation (PE) is a highly prevalent and complex syndrome that remains poorly defined and inadequately characterized. Pharmacotherapy represents the current basis of lifelong PE treatment.

Aim.—The goal of this study was to assess the role of phosphodiesterase type 5 inhibitors (PDE5-Is) in the treatment of patients with PE without associated erectile dysfunction (ED).

Main Outcome Measure.—The posttreatment intravaginal ejaculatory latency time was used as the primary end point of efficacy.

Methods.—A systematic review of the literature was performed by electronically searching the MedLine database for peer-reviewed articles regarding the mechanism of action and the clinical trials of PDE5 in the management of PE. A meta-analysis of these clinical studies was performed to pool the efficacy.

Results.—Twenty-nine articles that examined the supposed mechanisms of action and 14 articles that reported data from clinical studies were reviewed. The PDE5 may exert their influence by increasing the levels of nitric oxide both centrally (reducing sympathetic drive) and peripherally (leading to smooth-muscle dilatation of the seminal tract). These drugs may also induce peripheral analgesia to prolong the duration of the erection, increase confidence, improve the perception of ejaculatory control and overall sexual satisfaction, and decrease the postorgasmic refractory time for achieving a second erection after ejaculation. Concerning the efficacy, the meta-analysis shows an overall positive effect for the use of PDE5 as monotherapy or as components of a combination regimen in the treatment of PE. The major limitations of the published literature included poor study design, the absence of solid methodology, which was characterized by the lack of a unique PE definition, and the lack of appropriate endpoints for outcome evaluation of a placebo control arm and of Institutional Review Board approval.

Conclusion.—There is inadequate, partial basic, and clinical evidence to support the use of PDE5 for the treatment of PE.

▶ It is not surprising that PDE5 inhibitors are used for nearly every sort of sexual dysfunction in men. Despite being indicated only for the management of organic erectile dysfunction (ED), most providers have likely at least considered or actually prescribed these medications for psychogenic ED, hypoactive sexual desire disorder, delayed orgasm, Peyronie's disease, and/or premature ejaculation.

As ostensibly the most common male sexual disorder, premature ejaculation is likely the sexual dysfunction indication (other than ED) for which PDE5I are most often prescribed or researched. This meta-analytic review highlights mechanisms by which PDE5I may modulate the process of ejaculation as well as clinical trials of PDE5I for medical management of PE. There is evidence that these medications may be efficacious, perhaps for physiological reasons, both peripherally and centrally. It may also be hypothesized that enhancement in sexual confidence and ability to sustain erection may play an important role. It is likely that PDE5I will continue to play a role in PE management, at least until a therapy specifically approved for management of PE is widely available.

A. W. Shindel, MD

Long-Term Changes of Sexual Function in Men with Obstructive Sleep Apnea after Initiation of Continuous Positive Airway Pressure
Budweiser S, Luigart R, Jörres RA, et al (RoMed Clinical Ctr Rosenheim, Germany; Univ of Regensburg, Germany; Ludwig-Maximilians-Univ, Munich, Germany; et al)
J Sex Med 2012 [Epub ahead of print]

Introduction.—Obstructive sleep apnea (OSA), particularly intermittent nocturnal hypoxemia, is associated with erectile dysfunction (ED).

Aim.—We investigated in patients with OSA whether continuous positive airway pressure (CPAP) therapy has a long-term effect on sexual function, including ED, in the presence of other risk factors for ED.

Methods.—Within a long-term observational design, we reassessed 401 male patients who had been referred for polysomnography, with respect to erectile and overall sexual function. Mean ± standard deviation follow-up time was 36.5 ± 3.7 months. Patients with moderate to severe ED were stratified according to the regular use of CPAP.

Main Outcome Measure.—Changes of sexual function were assessed by the 15-item International Index of Erectile Function (IIEF-15) questionnaire, including the domains erectile function (EF), intercourse satisfaction, orgasmic function (OF), sexual desire (SD), and overall satisfaction (OS).

Results.—Of the 401 patients, 91 returned a valid IIEF-15 questionnaire at follow-up. Their baseline characteristics were not different from those of the total study group. OSA (apnea—hypopnea index > 5/hour) had been diagnosed in 91.2% of patients. In patients with moderate to severe ED (EF domain < 17), CPAP users (N = 21) experienced an improvement in overall sexual function (IIEF-15 summary score; $P = 0.014$) compared with CPAP non-users (N = 18), as well as in the subdomains OF ($P = 0.012$), SD ($P = 0.007$), and OS ($P = 0.033$). Similar results were obtained in patients with poor overall sexual dysfunction (IIEF-15 summary score < 44). In patients with moderate to severe ED and low mean nocturnal oxygen saturation (≤93%, median), also the EF subdomain improved in CPAP users vs. non-users ($P = 0.047$).

Conclusions.—These data indicate that long-term CPAP treatment of OSA and the related intermittent hypoxia can improve or preserve sexual function in men with OSA and moderate to severe erectile or sexual dysfunction, suggesting a certain reversibility of OSA-induced sexual dysfunctions.

▶ Sleep apnea is an increasingly common diagnosis and a preventable source of substantial morbidity. In this study with an unfortunately low level of participation (less than 25% response rate), men who were "regular" continuous positive airway pressure (CPAP) users experienced stability in their scores on all sub-domains of the International Index of Erectile Function (IIEF) compared with non-CPAP users, who were noted to have significant declines in sexual desire and overall satisfaction. Furthermore, those men with moderate-severe erectile dysfunction (ED) at baseline who used CPAP at follow-up had higher scores on the orgasmic satisfaction, sexual desire, and overall satisfaction domains of the IIEF compared with men with moderate-severe ED who did not use CPAP. The authors also report a higher "composite" measure of sexual function in men as assessed by the IIEF-total, a metric that is in my mind of unclear validity; each individual domain of the IIEF assesses a specific part of sexual function in men, but does the composite score have a particular meaning? No reference is supplied to provide support for the author's categorization of different scores for IIEF composite as "good," "fair," or "poor."

This is an interesting report by virtue of the prevalence of obstructive sleep apnea and its long follow-up period. However, methodological limitations complicate interpretation of results. Subgroup analysis of men with moderate to severe ED is also somewhat methodologically dubious; with enough data-mining and parsing of data, it is nearly always possible to produce "significant" results. A clearer statement of primary and secondary outcome measures and power analysis to determine appropriateness of sample size are 2 important features that this study lacks. Hopefully this article will be a stimulus toward better designed studies of the intersection between ED and obstructive sleep apnea.

A. W. Shindel, MD

The Role of Initial Success Rates and Other Factors in Determining Reliability of Outcomes of Phosphodiesterase Inhibitor Therapy for Erectile Dysfunction: A Pooled Analysis of 17 Placebo-Controlled Trials of Tadalafil for Use as Needed

Sontag A, Rosen RC, Litman HJ, et al (Eli Lilly and Company, Indianapolis, IN; New England Res Insts, Inc, Watertown, MA)
J Sex Med 2012 [Epub ahead of print]

Introduction.—Reliability of successful outcomes in men with erectile dysfunction (ED) on phosphodiesterase type 5 inhibitors is an important aspect of patient management.

Aims.—We examined reliability of successful outcomes in a large integrated dataset of randomized tadalafil trials.

Main Outcome Measures.—Success rates, time to success, subsequent success after first success, and probability of success were analyzed based on Sexual Encounter Profile questions 2 and 3.

Methods.—Data from 3,254 ED patients treated with tadalafil 10 mg (N = 510), 20 mg (N = 1,772), or placebo (N = 972) were pooled from 17 placebo-controlled studies.

Results.—Tadalafil patients had significantly higher first-attempt success rates vs. placebo. This effect was consistent across most subgroups; however, patients with severe ED experienced a greater response to tadalafil than patients with mild–moderate ED. Approximately 80% of patients achieved successful penile insertion within two attempts with either tadalafil dose and successful intercourse within eight attempts for tadalafil 10 mg and four attempts for tadalafil 20 mg. However, approximately 70% of tadalafil-treated patients achieved successful intercourse even by the second attempt. Subsequent success rates were higher for patients with first-attempt success (81.5% for 10 mg and 86.1% for 20 mg vs. 66.2% for placebo, $P < 0.001$) vs. patients with later initial success (53.2% for 10 mg and 56.4% for 20 mg vs. 39.9% for placebo, $P < 0.001$). Among patients treated with tadalafil, intercourse success rates at early attempts were similar to rates at later attempts (i.e., attempts 5 and 10 vs. 25), although insertion success rates were significantly lower earlier in treatment.

Conclusions.—The findings affirm the reliability of successful outcomes with tadalafil treatment and that first-attempt success is a critical factor affecting subsequent outcomes. The results further show that even among men who did not succeed on first attempt, a substantial proportion will have successful outcomes if treatment is maintained.

▶ Despite established efficacy at the population level, many men fail management with PDE5 inhibitors. This may be due to severity of comorbid disease states; however, it may also be the case that some men do not experience initial success when using the drug for the first time and become frustrated or depressed. Despite their power, PDE5Is are very dependent on state of mind and sexual arousal, and it is logical to hypothesize that men who approach their use with trepidation, worry, or generally low sexual confidence will oftentimes fail because of their psychological state.

All providers encounter patients who return to the office after having received an ED medication with the report that "it didn't work." In many of these cases, patients have taken the medication incorrectly or tried just once and then given up. These data indicate that a fair number of men may need more than one attempt to achieve success when using PDE5 inhibitors. This point needs to be emphasized to patients at first prescription; providers should do everything they can to help the patient have a first-use success as this is obviously a very important determinant of whether or not the pills will work long-term. This includes providing instructions on proper use (eg, food intake, appropriate dosing interval, need for sexual stimulation).

A. W. Shindel, MD

Internet-Ordered Viagra (Sildenafil Citrate) Is Rarely Genuine
Campbell N, Clark JP, Stecher VJ, et al (Pfizer Inc, NY; et al)
J Sex Med 9:2943-2951, 2012

Introduction.—Counterfeit medication is a growing problem. This study assessed the requirement for prescription, cost, origin, and content of medications sold via the Internet and purporting to be the phosphodiesterase type 5 inhibitor Viagra (sildenafil citrate).

Methods.—Pfizer monitored top search results for the query "buy Viagra" on the two leading Internet search engines in March 2011. Orders were placed from 22 unique Web sites claiming to sell Viagra manufactured by Pfizer. Tablets received were assessed for chemical composition.

Results.—No Web site examined required a prescription for purchase or a health screening survey; 90% offered illegal "generic Viagra." Cost per tablet ranged from $3.28–$33.00. Shipment origins of purchases were Hong Kong (N = 11), the United States (N = 6), and the United Kingdom (N = 2) as well as Canada, China, and India (N = 1 each). Notably, the four Internet pharmacies claiming to be Canadian did not ship medication from a Canadian address. Of 22 sample tablets examined, 17 (77%) were counterfeit, 4 (18%) were authentic, and 1 (5%) was an illegal generic. Counterfeit tablets were analyzed for sildenafil citrate, the active pharmaceutical ingredient (API) of Viagra, and contents varied between 30% and 50% of the label claim. Counterfeits lacked product information leaflets, including appropriate safety warnings, and genuine Viagra formulations.

Conclusion.—Internet sites claiming to sell authentic Viagra shipped counterfeit medication 77% of the time; counterfeits usually came from non-U.S. addresses and had 30% to 50% of the labeled API claim. Caution is warranted when purchasing Viagra via the Internet.

▶ The sad fact remains that many men are hesitant to discuss sexuality and sexual dysfunction with their health care providers. The advent of the Internet makes it easy for these men to seek help anonymously; unfortunately, it also makes them subject to predatory business practices of businesses all too eager to take advantage of embarrassment and insecurity regarding sex.

This is an important study because it objectively shows that many of the products sold online, such as Viagra, are, in fact, counterfeit and contain variable amounts of the active ingredient; other studies have found that a fair number of these drugs may also contain contaminants.

It is useful for doctors to know this information and to caution their patients about the dangers of online purchasing from pharmacies not regulated by the US Food and Drug Administration or a similar body. At a minimum, pharmacies should require a prescription for purchase (none of these pharmacies did). Unfortunately, the (likely) large number of patients who do not see their doctors about sexual concerns will not hear this message there; clearly, public health efforts will also be required to promote awareness of the risks of ordering from nonregulated pharmacies and dispensaries. Finally, efforts and means to reduce the high cost of prescription drugs might help dissuade men from gambling on Internet-ordered drugs.

A. W. Shindel, MD

Quality of life in women with vulvar cancer submitted to surgical treatment: a comparative study

de Melo Ferreira AP, de Figueiredo EM, Lima RA, et al (Paulista State Univ, Botucatu, São Paulo, Brazil; Universidade Federal de Minas Gerais, Belo Horizonte, Brazil; et al)

Eur J Obstet Gynecol Reprod Biol 165:91-95, 2012

Objectives.—To investigate the occurrence and severity of lymphoedema of the lower extremities (LLE), quality of life (QoL), and urinary and sexual dysfunction in women with vulvar cancer submitted to surgical treatment.

Study Design.—Twenty-eight patients with vulvar cancer submitted to vulvectomy and inguinofemoral lymphadenectomy and 28 healthy, age-matched women (control group) were evaluated. The occurrence and severity of LLE were determined by Miller's Clinical Evaluation. QoL, urinary function and sexual function were assessed by the EORTC QLQ-C30, SF-ICIQ and FSFI questionnaires, respectively. The differences between groups and correlations were assessed using Student's t-test, Chi-squared test, Mann—Whitney U-test and Spearman's rho test.

Results.—The groups were similar in terms of marital status, educational status, menopausal status, hormone therapy and height. The occurrence and severity of LLE were higher in women with vulvar cancer compared with the control group ($p < 0.001$ and $p = 0.003$, respectively). A significant association was found between the severity of LLE and advanced age ($p = 0.04$), and the severity of LLE and higher body mass index (BMI; $p = 0.04$) in patients with vulvar cancer. In the patients with vulvar cancer, there was a significant correlation between the severity of LLE and worse QoL in the following domains: physical, cognitive, emotional, social, fatigue, pain, sleep and financial questions ($p < 0.05$). There was no difference in urinary function between the two groups ($p = 0.113$). Age and number of deliveries were the only variables associated with the occurrence of urinary incontinence ($p = 0.01$). Urinary incontinence was present in women with a mean age of 74.9 ± 4.6 years and a mean of 7.3 ± 1.3 normal deliveries. There was no difference between the groups in terms of the sexual function. Multivariate analysis showed an association between sexual function and age ($p = 0.01$), and sexual function and being in a stable relationship ($p = 0.02$).

Conclusion.—Patients submitted to vulvectomy or inguinofemoral lymphadenectomy for vulvar cancer are at higher risk of developing LLE compared with healthy, age-matched women. This has a negative effect on QoL, but does not interfere with urinary or sexual function.

▶ This article is an interesting example of how the notion that vulvar cancer does not interfere with sexual function can be promulgated when practitioners do not read beyond the abstract. The authors state that there is no difference in sexual function between women who have and have not undergone vulvectomy for cancer. This is a somewhat difficult statement to reconcile with such an aggressive surgical intervention.

Upon closer reading, it is clear that this study's primary endpoint is lower extremity lymphedema; sexual function is assessed using only the Female Sexual Function Index (FSFI) in the absence of any other clear assessment of sexual function. Just 21% of the patients and 32% of the controls (6 and 9 patients, respectively) had an active sexual life, although what this implies and how it was assessed is unclear. The authors report individual FSFI domains, and there are relatively large differences between the mean scores for the domains of interest. Of course, one must ask if a population of 15 subjects is adequate power to detect a clinically relevant difference in sexual function. To their credit, the authors acknowledge the limitations of such a limited set of sexual function data, but this text is buried near the end of the discussion section where many readers will not look.

This article is selected not because of its merit but rather as a cautionary example. The authors have potentially done harm by stating, with such unequivocal certainty and based on such flimsy data, that vulvar surgery does not impact sexual function.

A. W. Shindel, MD

The Impact of Androgen Receptor CAG Repeat Polymorphism on Andropausal Symptoms in Different Serum Testosterone Levels
Liu C-C, Lee Y-C, Wang C-J, et al (Kaohsiung Med Univ Hosp, Taiwan; et al)
J Sex Med 9:2429-2437, 2012

Introduction.—In addition to a depletion of androgen, attenuated action of androgen receptor (AR) might also contribute to andropausal symptoms.

Aim.—To evaluate the interaction of AR cytosine adenine guanine (CAG) repeat polymorphism and serum testosterone levels and their effect on andropausal symptoms in aging Taiwanese men.

Methods.—From August 2007 to April 2008, a free health screening for men older than 40 years was conducted by a medical center in Kaohsiung City, Taiwan. All participants received physical examination, answered questionnaires to collect their demographic information and medical histories, completed the Androgen Deficiency in the Aging Male (ADAM) questionnaire, and provided 20-cm^3 whole blood samples for biochemical and genetic evaluation.

Main Outcome Measures.—The ADAM questionnaire was used to evaluate andropausal symptoms. Serum albumin, total testosterone (TT), and sex hormone-binding globulin levels were measured. Free testosterone level was calculated. AR gene CAG repeat polymorphism was determined by direct sequencing.

Results.—Seven hundred two men with the mean age of 57.2 ± 6.5 years were included. There was no significant association between TT levels and the distribution of AR CAG repeat polymorphism. When TT levels were above 340 ng/dL, subjects with AR CAG repeat lengths ≧25 showed significantly higher risk of developing andropausal symptoms, as compared with those with AR CAG repeat lengths ≤ 22 ($P = 0.006$), but this was not observed when TT levels were 340 ng/dL or below. Age and number of comorbidities were also independent risk factors for andropausal symptoms.

Conclusion.—In subjects with normal TT concentration, those with longer AR CAG repeat lengths have a higher risk of developing andropausal symptoms. Age and number of comorbidities can also influence the appearance of andropausal symptoms. In clinical practice, a multifactorial approach to evaluate andropausal symptoms and the interactions between those risk factors is suggested.

▶ This fascinating and important study takes us beyond the admittedly imperfect metric of total (and even bioavailable) testosterone as a metric to determine at what level testosterone supplementation may be beneficial. Clearly, testosterone itself is of little import without activation of the androgen receptor, and it is well known that cytosine adenine guanine (CAG) repeat length plays an important role in modulating androgen receptor activity. In this study, men with long CAG repeat lengths had increased risk of hypogonadal symptoms compared with men with shorter repeats even if testosterone was greater than 340 ng/dL. This difference was not significant in those men whose levels were already less than 340 ng/dL.

The authors used the Androgen Deficiency in the Aging Male (ADAM) questionnaire, which despite its limitations is one of the more commonly used screeners for symptoms possibly related to hypogonadism. By ADAM criteria, most of these men had symptoms of hypogonadism; this may be a factor of age, the general vagueness of the ADAM questionnaire, or that subjects were recruited from a health screening.

Despite this limitation, this is very exciting work that may help us better understand why some men may endorse symptoms of hypogonadism, even with normal serum testosterone levels, and others may feel well at lower levels of testosterone. CAG repeat length is not at this time a clinically useful or available test, but this may change with further research.

A. W. Shindel, MD

WNT2 Locus Is Involved in Genetic Susceptibility of Peyronie's Disease

Dolmans GH, Werker PM, de Jong IJ, et al (Univ Med Ctr Groningen and Univ of Groningen, the Netherlands; et al)

J Sex Med 9:1430-1434, 2012

Introduction.—Peyronie's disease (PD) is a fibromatosis of the penis, with a pathology very similar to what is seen in the hand (palmar fascia) in Dupuytren's disease (DD). Recently, we performed a genome-wide association study and identified nine genetic loci containing common variants associated with DD. Seven of these loci mapped within or near genes of the canonical WNT pathway and each locus yielded relatively large odds ratios (ORs) for DD disease status.

Aim.—Given the clinical overlap between PD and DD, we examined whether the nine DD susceptibility loci are also involved in PD.

Methods.—An association study was performed using a case/control design. From 2007 to 2010, we prospectively included 111 men who had been clinically diagnosed with PD. Control subjects (N = 490 males) were randomly drawn from a population-based cohort from the same region of the Netherlands. Allele frequencies in the 111 PD cases and 490 controls were compared using a 1-degree-of-freedom basic chi-square test. A *P* value < 0.05 after Bonferroni correction for the nine tested single nucleotide polymorphisms (SNPs) was considered statistically significant (i.e., *P* < 0.0056).

Main Outcome Measure.—Association of genetic markers (SNPs) with PD.

Results.—We observed significant association with SNP rs4730775 at the wingless-type MMTV integration site family member 2 (*WNT2*) locus on chromosome 7 (*P* = 0.0015, OR 0.61), but found no evidence for the other eight loci being involved with PD despite the large effect size seen for some of these variants in DD. The *WNT2* association was even more significant after we removed 15 patients with comorbid DD.

Conclusions.—*WNT2* is a susceptibility locus for PD and our finding provides evidence for a partly shared genetic susceptibility between PD and DD.

▶ It is fairly well established that Peyronie disease has a genetic component and is associated with other abnormalities of collagen metabolism. This case-control study reports a single nucleotide polymorphism (SNP) modulating expression of the *WNT2* gene that was significantly associated with presence of the Peyronie phenotype; this SNP had been previously associated with Dupuytren contractures so likely plays a role in a variety of collagen healing disorders. *WNT2* encodes glycoproteins that have roles in stimulating cell proliferation and survival, 2 characteristics that are very much involved in development of the Peyronie's phenotype.

The study is slightly limited in that the Dupuytren or Peyronie status of the control population is unknown. Despite this, it is an exciting breakthrough in our understanding of the biological underpinnings of Peyronie disease.

A. W. Shindel, MD

Incomplete Recovery of Erectile Function in Rat after Discontinuation of Dual 5-Alpha Reductase Inhibitor Therapy

Öztekin ÇV, Gur S, Abdulkadir NA, et al (Ankara Numune Education and Res Hosp, Turkey; Ankara Univ School of Pharmacy, Turkey; et al)
J Sex Med 9:1773-1781, 2012

Aim.—The association of 5-alpha reductase inhibitor (5ARI) therapy and sexual dysfunction has been reported. Some patients claim persistent erectile dysfunction despite long-term discontinuation of 5ARI treatment. The aim of this study was to assess erectile function after cessation of 5ARI therapy using a rat model.

Methods.—Twenty-six adult male Sprague-Dawley rats were randomized into three groups: (i) control (N = 10); (ii) 8-week dutasteride treatment (0.5 mg/rat/day, in drinking water, N = 8); and (iii) 6-week dutasteride treatment followed by a 2-week washout period (N = 8). The experiments were performed after 8 weeks from the initiation of treatment in all groups. In vivo erectile activity and in vitro contractile and relaxant responses of cavernosal smooth muscle were investigated.

Results.— In vivo erectile activity (intracavernosal pressure [ICP]/mean arterial pressure [MAP] and total ICP) in treatment groups were significantly decreased compared with controls (ICP/MAP: $P < 0.001$ for 2.5 v, 5 v, and 7.5 v; total ICP: $P < 0.001$ for 5 v and $P < 0.01$ for 7.5 v). Acetylcholine-induced relaxations were diminished in treatment groups ($P < 0.05$). Relaxant responses to electrical field stimulation (EFS) were decreased in the 8-week treatment group ($P < 0.05$) but were similar to controls in the washout group. Sodium nitroprusside (SNP)-induced endothelium-independent relaxations were reduced in the 8-week dutasteride treatment group ($P < 0.01$), while these responses were restored in the washout group. The contractile responses to the alpha1-adrenergic agonist phenylephrine were decreased in treatment groups compared with controls ($P < 0.01$). Direct neurogenic contractile responses in the dutasteride groups were significantly lower than controls between 1 and 15 Hz frequencies (but not at 20 Hz) and washout partially restored the responses at 10 and 15 Hz.

Conclusion.—Discontinuation of dutasteride improved the relaxant responses to EFS and SNP, while cholinergic and adrenergic responses remained depressed. Our findings suggest a time dependent detriment of dutasteride on erectile function. The withdrawal/washout effect of 5ARIs on parameters of human sexual function warrants further investigation.

▶ A great deal of emotion surrounds the debate concerning if and how 5-alpha reductase inhibitors (ARI) may contribute to persistent sexual dysfunction. There are several clinical publications, numerous Web sites, and several physiology review articles that highlight ways in which 5ARI may exert a negative effect on male sexual function. Despite this, the mechanisms by which 5ARI impair sexual function remain a mystery.

This article is a welcome addition to our knowledge base of how 5ARI impact sexual function in a model animal system. In this study, it was demonstrated that in vivo erectile response to cavernous nerve stimulation was depressed in animals that were treated with dutasteride for 8 weeks or for 6 weeks with a 2-week washout period. Interestingly, organ bath studies indicated that washout of dutasteride was associated with normalization of cavernous tissue response to electrical field stimulation and sodium nitroprusside; however, the response to cholinergic and adrenergic stimuli remained depressed. It is implied that persistent negative effects of dutasteride on erectile function may be related to changes in the autonomic innervations of the penis. This finding is all the more interesting as cholinergic responses facilitate, and adrenergic responses inhibit, erections. Clearly, more research is needed to sort out this complex physiology.

A. W. Shindel, MD

Estrogens in Men: Clinical Implications for Sexual Function and the Treatment of Testosterone Deficiency

Kacker R, Traish AM, Morgentaler A (Harvard Med School, Boston, MA; Boston Univ, MA)

J Sex Med 9:1681-1696, 2012

Introduction.—The role of estrogens in male sexual function and the pathogenesis of testosterone deficiency remain controversial and poorly understood.

Aims.—To review the distribution of estrogens in normal and testosterone deficient men, their potential role in sexual function, and the clinical implications of elevated estrogens during testosterone therapy.

Methods.—A comprehensive, broad-based literature review was conducted on the role of estrogens in male sexual function and testosterone deficiency.

Results.—Estrogens elicit a variety of physiological responses in men and may contribute to modulation of sexual function. In the absence of testosterone deficiency, elevations in estrogens do not appear to be harmful and estrogens may help maintain some, but not all, sexual function in castrated men. While the therapeutic use of estrogens at pharmacologic doses has been used to suppress serum testosterone, naturally occurring elevations of estrogens do not appear to be a cause of low testosterone. During testosterone replacement, estrogens may rise and occasionally reach elevated levels. There is a lack of evidence that treatment of elevated estrogen levels during testosterone replacement has benefit in terms of male sexuality.

Conclusion.—Further research on the importance of estrogens in male sexual function is needed. Current evidence does not support a role of naturally occurring estrogen elevations in testosterone deficiency or the treatment of elevated estrogens during testosterone therapy.

▶ Testosterone and estrogen are colloquially known as "the male" and "the female" hormone, respectively. This oversimplification ignores the fact that people of either gender produce both hormones, albeit in markedly different quantities. Given the assumed gender specificity of each hormone, it is not surprising that many patients and providers attribute negative attributes to actions of the "opposite-gendered" hormone in patients. This is likely a fallacy, because testosterone in appropriate quantities has been clearly associated with positive effects on sexual function and some other parameters in women.

This review attempts to dissect the potentially positive actions of estrogens in men. There is good evidence that estrogen may be important in bone health and skeletal development and cardiovascular function. The data on estrogen's role in male sexual function remain controversial; there is abundant evidence (albeit of mixed quality) that estrogens may exert negative effects on sexual function. However, scattered reports from populations of men (particularly those with low testosterone) suggest that estrogen may play a salvage role in preserving sexual function. These data are weak but intriguing. It is clear that a more nuanced approach to research and assessment of estrogen's role in male sexuality is needed.

A. W. Shindel, MD

Cyclic AMP-dependent phosphorylation of neuronal nitric oxide synthase mediates penile erection

Hurt KJ, Sezen SF, Lagoda GF, et al (Univ of Colorado Anschutz Med Campus, Aurora; The Julius Hopkins Univ School of Medicine, Baltimore, MD; et al)
Proc Natl Acad Sci U S A 109:16624-16629, 2012

Nitric oxide (NO) generated by neuronal NO synthase (nNOS) initiates penile erection, but has not been thought to participate in the sustained erection required for normal sexual performance. We now show that cAMP-dependent phosphorylation of nNOS mediates erectile physiology, including sustained erection. nNOS is phosphorylated by cAMP-dependent protein kinase (PKA) at serine(S)1412. Electrical stimulation of the penile innervation increases S1412 phosphorylation that is blocked by PKA inhibitors but not by PI3-kinase/Akt inhibitors. Stimulation of cAMP formation by forskolin also activates nNOS phosphorylation. Sustained penile erection elicited by either intracavernous forskolin injection, or augmented by forskolin during cavernous nerve electrical stimulation, is prevented by the NOS inhibitor L-NAME, or in nNOS-deleted mice. Thus, nNOS mediates both initiation and maintenance of penile erection, implying unique approaches for treating erectile dysfunction.

▶ The conventional teaching on penile erection is that nitric oxide (NO) derived from nNOS provides the spark for erection via entry of calcium into smooth muscle cells. Subsequent shear forces on endothelial tissue stimulate eNOS to sustain NO production. These authors demonstrate that electrical stimulation of cavernous nerves leads to phosphorylation of nNOS and enhancement of activity for this enzyme. This effect appears to be mediated by action of protein kinase A (PKA) and appears to be sustained after penile erection; one can deduce from this that nNOS remains a potential contributor to production of NO and hence penile erection even after erection initiation.

This study does not do much to immediately revolutionize the medical management of erectile dysfunction. However, the net result of their various findings is that novel drugs that inhibit metabolism of cAMP and cGMP may have a synergistic effect in directly enhancing NO production, which will in turn further enhance production of cGMP. Such drugs may have a place in erectile dysfunction treatment for the future.

A. W. Shindel, MD

The Effects of Hormonal Contraceptives on Female Sexuality: A Review
Burrows LJ, Basha M, Goldstein AT (The Ctr for Vulvar and Vaginal Disorders, Akron, OH; Georgetown Univ, Washington, DC; The Ctr for Vulvovaginal Disorders, Washington, DC)
J Sex Med 9:2213-2223, 2012

Introduction.—Hormonal contraceptives can influence female sexual function.

Aim.—The goal of this article was to provide a comprehensive review of the effects that various hormonal contraceptives may have on female sexual function.

Methods.—A Medline search was conducted using several terms related to and including the terms contraception, oral contraceptive, female sexual function, dyspareunia, libido, and sexual desire.

Results.—A thorough review of the effects of hormonal contraceptives on female sexual function.

Conclusions.—The sexual side effects of hormonal contraceptives are not well studied, particularly with regard to impact on libido. There appears to be mixed effects on libido, with a small percentage of women experiencing an increase or a decrease, and the majority being unaffected. Healthcare providers must be aware that hormonal contraceptive can have negative effects on female sexuality so they can counsel and care for their patients appropriately.

▶ This article would perhaps be more useful in a contraception or obstetric/gynecologic journal, but it's an important topic that any provider interested in sexual health should consider. Do oral contraceptive pills contribute to sexual dysfunction in women?

In my opinion, a woman has the right to enjoy sexual activity and simultaneously have control over if and when she becomes pregnant. Effective and easy-to-use contraception is of critical importance in support of this right, and hormonal contraceptives, particularly oral contraceptive pills, play an essential role. As with any other medical intervention, hormonal manipulation does carry some risks. The potential vascular and neoplastic effects of hormonal contraceptives are generally discussed with patients, but many providers may be unaware and/or choose to ignore potential sexual side effects of hormone manipulation in women.

It is evident from the published data that many women use hormonal contraceptives with no observed ill effects. Indeed, some women report enhancement of sexual response. This may be related to security regarding control of pregnancy status or other mechanisms. It is also evident that some women experience bothersome sexual side effects after initiation of hormonal contraception, specifically decreased vaginal lubrication, decreased libido, dyspareunia, and possibly tissue changes in the vagina and labia. Providers who supply contraceptives to women should counsel patients on these risks and provide alternative management strategies (eg, barrier methods, intrauterine devices, natural family planning) options for women who experience bothersome sexual side effects.

A. W. Shindel, MD

Safety and Efficacy of Once Daily Administration of 50 mg Mirodenafil in Patients with Erectile Dysfunction: a Multicenter, Double-Blind, Placebo Controlled Trial

Chung JH, Kang DH, Oh CY, et al (Hanyang Univ College of Medicine, Seoul, Korea; Hallym Univ, Chuncheon, Korea; et al)

J Urol 189:1006-1013, 2013

Purpose.—We evaluated the improvement in erectile dysfunction and lower urinary tract symptoms as well as the safety of once daily administration of 50 mg mirodenafil in men with erectile dysfunction.

Materials and Methods.—A total of 226 patients visited for treatment of erectile dysfunction and were recruited for the study. Of these men 180 met the study inclusion criteria after completing a 2-week screening period (visit [V]1). The patients were randomly allocated into 2 groups. Group 1 (90 patients) received 50 mg mirodenafil once daily and group 2 (90 patients) received a placebo daily. Blood pressure, heart rate, IIEF-5 (5-item version of the International Index of Erectile Function), and SEP (Sexual Encounter Profile) questions 2 and 3 were assessed at 4 (V2), 8 (V3) and 12 weeks after the start of treatment (V4). I-PSS (International Prostate Symptom Score), maximal flow rate and post-void residual volume were also assessed for the evaluation of lower urinary tract symptoms.

Results.—Of the 180 patients 71 in group 1 and 63 in group 2 completed the 12-week clinical trial. IIEF-5 and I-PSS significantly improved in group 1 ($p < 0.001$ for both). Facial flushing was the most common adverse effect, followed by headaches. Notably there were no statistically significant differences in either of the variables related to the cardiovascular system.

Conclusions.—Once daily administration of 50 mg mirodenafil was efficacious and safe for the treatment of erectile dysfunction and lower urinary tract symptoms.

▶ The 3 phosphodiesterase type 5 inhibitors (PDE5I) that are commercially available in the United States are not the only PDE5I currently used around the world for treatment of erectile dysfunction (ED). A number of other drugs from this family have been approved for use in other countries. This particular study reports on mirodenafil, one of several PDE5Is developed and used in South Korea. Interestingly, this study looked at a daily dose option, currently only approved for use with tadalafil. Mirodenafil was found to be efficacious in treatment of ED and lower urinary tract symptoms with a reasonable side effect profile. Most interestingly, in this study, treatment with the drug was found to be associated with improved urine flow rate, an objective finding not well identified in prior studies of daily dose tadalafil.

In a strange and not well explained additional investigation, the authors reported on response to the Premature Ejaculation Diagnostic Tool (PEDT), a validated instrument for assessment of PE. The mean PEDT score for both groups at baseline was 10, suggesting probable PE. They do not address the PEDT in any particular detail during the methods or results section; indeed, they don't even cite the validation study for this instrument; it seems almost an afterthought. That said, the placebo arm in this study experienced an explicable increase in their PEDT score, suggesting that many men taking placebo went on to have distressingly rapid ejaculation. The mechanism or meaning behind this is hard to understand.

Despite the strangeness of the PE assessment, a daily-dose medication for ED is attractive to some men as an option, particularly when there is the potential for concomitant improvement in bothersome urinary tract symptoms. This medication offers the additional advantage of leading to demonstrable changes in urodynamic parameters, an observation not found in other studies of PDE5I for lower urinary tract symptoms.

A. W. Shindel, MD

A Prospective Longitudinal Survey of Erectile Dysfunction in Patients with Localized Prostate Cancer Treated with Permanent Prostate Brachytherapy

Matsushima M, Kikuchi E, Maeda T, et al (Keio Univ School of Medicine, Tokyo, Japan; et al)
J Urol 189:1014-1018, 2013

Purpose.—Few studies have evaluated changes in erectile function with time before and after prostate brachytherapy using the International Index of Erectile Function-15, a sensitive, validated tool for assessing male sexual dysfunction. In this prospective study we evaluated the natural history of erectile function after prostate brachytherapy without supplemental therapy (external beam radiotherapy, phosphodiesterase-5 inhibitors or androgen deprivation therapy) using the International Index of Erectile Function-15.

Materials and Methods.—We identified 119 patients who were followed at least 12 months after prostate brachytherapy between 2004 and 2010. Sexual and erectile function status were assessed before brachytherapy (baseline), and 3, 6, 12, 18, 24 and 36 months postoperatively using the International Index of Erectile Function-15.

Results.—Mean total International Index of Erectile Function-15 score, and scores on the erectile function, orgasmic function, sexual desire and intercourse satisfaction domains 3 months after brachytherapy were significantly lower than at baseline ($p < 0.05$). They remained lower until 36 months after prostate brachytherapy. Erectile function was maintained 12 months after brachytherapy in 16 of the 48 men (33.3%) with a baseline erectile function domain score of 11 or greater. There was no significant difference in clinical features except the age of patients who maintained the erectile function domain score and their counterparts 12 months after brachytherapy. Multivariate analysis revealed that age 70 years or greater was the only predictive factor for deteriorating erectile function after brachytherapy ($p = 0.035$).

Conclusions.—Findings indicate a global decrease in all domains of the International Index of Erectile Function-15 score 12 months after prostate brachytherapy. Also, patient age may influence the preservation of brachytherapy related potency.

▶ This study of brachytherapy outcomes is of shorter duration than the study of Buckstein but benefits from more robust assessment of comorbidity and more precise metrics for assessment of erectile difficulty. Despite the fact that this study enrolls a much smaller population of patients (the majority of whom had some degree of erectile dysfunction [ED] per the International Index of Erectile Function [IIEF] survey), it remains a more useful study because of its inclusion of comorbidities, more stringent means of assessing ED, and inclusion of metrics to assess other domains of male sexual response.

The authors report that a third of men with no ED (IIEF-EF > 26 of 30) at baseline (n = 48) remained potent 12 months after treatment. They also come to the same conclusion as Buckstein in that age is an important predictor of worse erectile function outcomes over the long term; indeed, only age remained associated in multivariable analysis. It must be borne in mind, however, that this represents a relatively small subset of 48 patients.

A. W. Shindel, MD

Periprostatic Implantation of Human Bone Marrow-derived Mesenchymal Stem Cells Potentiates Recovery of Erectile Function by Intracavernosal Injection in a Rat Model of Cavernous Nerve Injury

You D, Jang MJ, Lee J, et al (Univ of Ulsan College of Medicine, Seoul, Korea; Asan Med Ctr, Seoul, Korea; Pharmicell Co. Ltd, Seoul, Korea; et al)
Urology 81:104-110, 2013

Objective.—To evaluate whether periprostatic implantation (PPI) of human bone marrow-derived mesenchymal stem cells (hBMSCs) potentiates recovery of erectile function after intracavernosal injection (ICI) of hBMSCs in a rat model of cavernous nerve (CN) injury.

Methods.—Sprague-Dawley rats that had undergone bilateral CN injury were treated by ICI with or without PPI of hBMSCs (10 rats per group). hBMSCs were harvested from healthy human donors. Fibrin scaffolds were used for PPI of hBMSCs. After 4 weeks, erectile responses to electric pelvic ganglion stimulation were studied. The expression of neuronal nitric oxide synthase (nNOS)-positive nerve fibers and smooth muscle/collagen ratio was evaluated in each penis.

Results.—ICI of hBMSCs slightly improved erectile function compared with the control group (maximal intracavernosal pressure/mean arterial pressure, 39.1% vs 21.7%; $P = .060$), but a combination of PPI and ICI significantly improved erectile function (45.0%, $P = .007$). After stem cell therapy, the number of nNOS-positive nerve fibers increased significantly in the PPI + ICI group ($P = .017$). The smooth muscle/collagen ratio increased significantly after stem cell therapy in the ICI and PPI + ICI groups (both $P < .001$).

Conclusion.—ICI of hBMSCs in a rat model of CN injury results in recovery of penile erection by decreasing corporeal smooth muscle deterioration and collagen deposition. PPI of hBMSCs potentiates recovery of erectile function by ICI of hBMSCs via regeneration of nNOS-containing nerve fibers.

▶ This study represents another report of stem cell therapy as a means to improve impaired penile hemodynamics in a rat model of erectile dysfunction, in this case related to cavernous nerve crush. This report is unique in that in one arm of the study stem cells were implanted next to the prostate in addition to administration by intracavernous injection. Fibrin scaffolds were used to hold the stem cells in proximity to the cavernous nerves crush site. This approach has the theoretical benefit of applying additional cells near the site of injury.

Several prior reports have investigated penile injection of stem cells alone. This approach has emerged as a very promising treatment in preclinical studies. In this study, intracorporal injection alone led to only marginally better responses compared with the control arm.

Stem cells have been purported to have the capacity to migrate to sites of injury, including injured cavernous nerves, after intracorporal injection. Whether use of stem cell—impregnated fibrin scaffolds is an effective adjunct is an interesting question for further investigation by other teams.

A. W. Shindel, MD

Increased Sexual Health After Restored Genital Sensation in Male Patients with Spina Bifida or a Spinal Cord Injury: the TOMAX Procedure

Overgoor MLE, de Jong TPVM, Cohen-Kettenis PT, et al (Isala Clinic, Zwolle, The Netherlands; Univ Children's Hosp UMC Utrecht and AMC Amsterdam, The Netherlands; VU Univ Med Centre, Amsterdam, The Netherlands; et al)
J Urol 189:626-632, 2013

Purpose.—In this study we prospectively investigated the contribution of restored penile sensation to sexual health in patients with low spinal lesions.

Materials and Methods.—In 30 patients (18 with spina bifida, 12 with spinal cord injury, age range 13 to 55 years) with no penile sensation but good groin sensation the new TOMAX (TO MAX-imize sensation, sexuality and quality of life) procedure was performed. This involves microsurgical connection of the sensory ilioinguinal nerve to the dorsal nerve of the penis unilaterally. Extensive preoperative and postoperative neurological and psychological evaluations were made.

Results.—A total of 24 patients (80%) gained unilateral glans penis sensation. This was initially felt as groin sensation but transformed into real glans sensation in 11 patients (33%). These patients had better overall sexual function ($p = 0.022$) and increased satisfaction ($p = 0.004$). Although 13 patients (43%) maintained groin sensation, their satisfaction with sexuality was only slightly less than that of those with glans sensation. Improved sensations helped them manage urinary incontinence, thereby improving personal hygiene and independence. Most patients felt more complete and less handicapped with their penis now part of their body image. They also reported having more open and meaningful sexual relationships with their partners.

Conclusions.—Tactile and erogenous sensitivity was restored in the glans penis in patients with a low spinal lesion. This new sensation enhanced the quality of sexual functioning and satisfaction. The TOMAX procedure should become standard treatment for such patients.

▶ Spinal cord injury or maldevelopment is a devastating occurrence that can have profound influence on quality of life and health. The sexual health ramifications merit special consideration because many individuals with spinal cord injury are young, with years of sexual and/or reproductive potential impacted by resultant sexual and fertility dysfunction.

The authors of this very interesting report detail a means to partially restore genital sensation in a cohort of men with congenital or acquired lower spinal defects with resultant genital numbness. By grafting the ilioinguinal nerve to the dorsal penile nerve, a majority of men gained some tactile awareness of contact to their penis. This sensation was felt primarily in the distribution of the inguinal nerve, although a third of patients acquired some feeling within the glans penis itself. There was a trend toward more reflexogenic erections (in response to penile contact) postoperatively and mean sexual satisfaction scores were superior posttreatment.

Although by no means perfect, this treatment appears to offer some benefit to men with penile numbness from spinal lesion. More studies from other centers are required to further study and refine this technique.

A. W. Shindel, MD

A 2-Stage Genome-Wide Association Study to Identify Single Nucleotide Polymorphisms Associated With Development of Erectile Dysfunction Following Radiation Therapy for Prostate Cancer
Kerns SL, Stock R, Stone N, et al (Mount Sinai School of Medicine, NY; et al)
Int J Radiat Oncol Biol Phys 85:e21-e28, 2013

Purpose.—To identify single nucleotide polymorphisms (SNPs) associated with development of erectile dysfunction (ED) among prostate cancer patients treated with radiation therapy.

Methods and Materials.—A 2-stage genome-wide association study was performed. Patients were split randomly into a stage I discovery cohort

(132 cases, 103 controls) and a stage II replication cohort (128 cases, 102 controls). The discovery cohort was genotyped using Affymetrix 6.0 genome-wide arrays. The 940 top ranking SNPs selected from the discovery cohort were genotyped in the replication cohort using Illumina iSelect custom SNP arrays.

Results.—Twelve SNPs identified in the discovery cohort and validated in the replication cohort were associated with development of ED following radiation therapy (Fisher combined P values 2.1×10^{-5} to 6.2×10^{-4}). Notably, these 12 SNPs lie in or near genes involved in erectile function or other normal cellular functions (adhesion and signaling) rather than DNA damage repair. In a multivariable model including nongenetic risk factors, the odds ratios for these SNPs ranged from 1.6 to 5.6 in the pooled cohort. There was a striking relationship between the cumulative number of SNP risk alleles an individual possessed and ED status (Sommers' D P value $= 1.7 \times 10^{-29}$). A 1-allele increase in cumulative SNP score increased the odds for developing ED by a factor of 2.2 (P value $= 2.1 \times 10^{-19}$). The cumulative SNP score model had a sensitivity of 84% and specificity of 75% for prediction of developing ED at the radiation therapy planning stage.

Conclusions.—This genome-wide association study identified a set of SNPs that are associated with development of ED following radiation therapy. These candidate genetic predictors warrant more definitive validation in an independent cohort.

▶ This interesting report provides some preliminary data on means by which providers can more accurately estimate the odds of erectile dysfunction (ED) after definitive treatment of prostate cancer, in this case by radiation therapy. The authors used genechip technology to ascertain which single nucleotide polymorphisms (SNPs) were associated with development of ED after prostate irradiation. None of the individual SNPs was predictive; however, a composite of 12 SNPs identified in the pilot data set and confirmed in a validation set was a useful tool for categorizing men who did or did not develop ED.

Unfortunately, several radiation delivery mechanisms and doses were used, so results must be interpreted with some caution. Furthermore, a variety of instruments were used to assess ED (Mount Sinai Erectile Function Score [SHIM]), and ED was defined somewhat loosely. "Cases" were men with any posttreatment SHIM score less than 7 (severe ED), and controls were defined as men with SHIM scores greater than 16 with or without phosphodiesterase 5I. Because a SHIM score of 22 or greater is generally construed as no ED and a score of 17 to 21 typically represents mild ED, these loose criteria leave much to be desired.

Despite these limitations, the article remains quite interesting. Personalized medicine (diagnosis, treatment, and prognostication) based on an individual's specific genetic makeup offers tremendous potential but unique challenges, including medico-legal and privacy concerns. Further development of this technology must be accompanied by public discourse involving all stakeholders (ie, everyone) to establish how/when this information is to be used/released.

A. W. Shindel, MD

Molecular Analysis of Erection Regulatory Factors in Sickle Cell Disease Associated Priapism in the Human Penis

Lagoda G, Sezen SF, Cabrini MR, et al (Johns Hopkins Med Institutions, Baltimore, MD)
J Urol 189:762-768, 2013

Purpose.—Priapism is a vasculopathy that occurs in approximately 40% of patients with sickle cell disease. Mouse models suggest that dysregulated nitric oxide synthase and RhoA/ROCK signaling as well as increased oxidative stress may contribute to the mechanisms of sickle cell disease associated priapism. We examined changes in the protein expression of nitric oxide synthase and ROCK signaling pathways, and a source of oxidative stress, NADPH oxidase, in penile erectile tissue from patients with a priapism history etiologically related and unrelated to sickle cell disease.

Materials and Methods.—Human penile erectile tissue was obtained from 5 patients with sickle cell disease associated priapism and from 6 with priapism of other etiologies during nonemergent penile prosthesis surgery for erectile dysfunction or priapism management and urethroplasty. Tissue was also obtained from 5 control patients without a priapism history during penectomy for penile cancer. Samples were collected, immediately placed in cold buffer and then frozen in liquid nitrogen. The expression of phosphodiesterase 5, endothelial nitric oxide synthase, neuronal nitric oxide synthase, inducible nitric oxide synthase, RhoA, ROCK1, ROCK2, $p47^{phox}$, $p67^{phox}$, $gp91^{phox}$ and β-actin were determined by Western blot analysis. Nitric oxide was measured using the Griess reaction.

Results.—In the sickle cell disease group phosphodiesterase 5 ($p < 0.05$), endothelial nitric oxide synthase ($p < 0.01$) and RhoA ($p < 0.01$) expression was significantly decreased, while $gp91^{phox}$ expression ($p < 0.05$) was significantly increased compared to control values. In the nonsickle cell disease group endothelial nitric oxide synthase, ROCK1 and $p47^{phox}$ expression (each $p < 0.05$) was significantly decreased compared to control values. Total nitric oxide levels were not significantly different between the study groups.

Conclusions.—Mechanisms of sickle cell disease associated priapism in the human penis may involve dysfunctional nitric oxide synthase and ROCK signaling, and increased oxidative stress associated with NADPH oxidase mediated signaling.

▶ This basic science research paper compares penile tissues from men with sickle cell disease—induced priapism to tissues from men without priapism and from men with non-sickle cell—related priapism episodes. In tissues from both types of men with priapism, proteins from the RhoA/ROCK pathway were downregulated. The RhoA/ROCK pathway is a calcium sensitization pathway that tends to promote muscle contraction by preventing dephosphorylation of the myosin light chain. Ergo, lower RhoA/ROCK activity will tend to promote smooth muscle relaxation, vasodilation, and cavernous artery inflow, a situation that is obviously undesirable in the compartment syndrome situation of priapism. Dysregulation of nitric oxide signaling and oxidative stress may also play a role.

The immediate relevance of this report to practicing urologists may be minimal, but this article represents important progress. Acquisition of human tissue for priapism research is obviously difficult, and the authors are to be congratulated on their work. Both sickle cell disease and priapism remain poorly understood conditions despite their prevalence and potentially devastating sequelae. Any new knowledge carries some hope that improved treatments and preventive measures may be forthcoming.

A. W. Shindel, MD

Autonomic Nervous System Dysfunction in Lifelong Premature Ejaculation: Analysis of Heart Rate Variability
Zorba OU, Cicek Y, Uzun H, et al (Rize Univ, Turkey; Muğla Univ, Turkey; Ondokuz Mayis Univ, Samsun, Turkey; et al)
Urology 80:1283-1286, 2012

Objective.—To identify autonomic nervous dysfunction in patients with lifelong premature ejaculation.

Methods.—The study participants were 25 men with lifelong premature ejaculation and 25 healthy controls. The parameters of 24-hour heart rate variability that are influenced by the autonomic nervous system were compared between the men with lifelong premature ejaculation and the healthy controls.

Results.—The laboratory results of all patients were within normal limits, and no significant differences were found between the patients and the controls in age, body weight, and body mass index. A low-frequency signal that is influenced by the sympathetic system was increased in the patients ($P = .026$). Furthermore, a high-frequency signal that is influenced by the parasympathetic system was decreased in the patients ($P = .011$). Finally, the low frequency-to-high frequency ratio, an indicator of the balance between the two components of the autonomic nervous system, was increased in the patients ($P = .002$).

Conclusion.—To our knowledge, no study has investigated the influence of the autonomic nervous system on 24-hour heart rate variability in premature ejaculation. In the present study, sympathetic activity was increased in men with lifelong premature ejaculation; this overactivity might lead to lifelong premature ejaculation. Additional studies are required to reveal the possible alteration of the autonomic nervous system in premature ejaculation.

▶ This analysis investigates heart rate variability, a metric for autonomic nervous system function, in a population of men with lifelong premature ejaculation (PE) compared with men with ejaculation latency within a normal range. It was determined that sympathetic nervous system tone was higher and parasympathetic tone lower in the men with PE. Because seminal emission is under control of the sympathetic nervous system, it is plausible that hyperactivity of this component of the nervous system may enhance the likelihood of semen deposition in the posterior urethra with subsequent reflex seminal ejection, thus completing the ejaculation cycle.

Use of a Holter monitor to assess heart rate variability is a technique foreign to most urologists and many sexual medicine practitioners. It is, however, an interesting application of technology to a vexing problem in sexual medicine research and practice. The autonomic nervous system's role in PE is an interesting topic for consideration and research. Whether these findings can be manipulated to produce a therapeutic target for PE is unclear.

A. W. Shindel, MD

The Use of Tramadol "On demand" for Premature Ejaculation: A Systematic Review
Wong BLK, Malde S (Medway Maritime Hosp, Gillingham, UK)
Urology 81:98-103, 2013

Objective.—To determine the efficacy and safety of tramadol in the treatment of premature ejaculation (PE) by systematically reviewing the results of randomized controlled trials.

Materials and Methods.—All studies evaluating the efficacy of tramadol for the treatment of PE published in peer reviewed medical journals between 2006 and March 2012 were identified by searching for the keywords "premature ejaculation" and "tramadol" in the PubMed database. Only randomized controlled trials published in the English language were included.

Results.—A total of 5 articles, comprising 823 patients, met the inclusion criteria for further analysis. Overall, tramadol on-demand results in a significant improvement in mean intravaginal ejaculatory latency time and symptom scores compared with placebo and in an improvement in partner sexual satisfaction scores. The rate of short-term adverse effects is low.

Conclusion.—Tramadol is an effective treatment for patients with PE and represents a promising alternative to the currently used oral pharmacologic agents. Longer-term safety studies, and those comparing tramadol with the selective serotonin receptor inhibitors, are essential to determine the place of tramadol in the treatment of this distressing condition.

▶ Tramadol has been reported as an efficacious management for premature ejaculation (PE) in a number of clinical articles. However, it is not currently recommended as a first-line therapy in the management of PE by most leading sexual medicine organizations. Generally, it is recommended that PE management be initiated with selective serotonin reuptake inhibitor, topical anesthetics, and/or psychobehavioral interventions.

This article summarizes the existing data on randomized controlled clinical trials of tramadol in the management of PE. Five studies were identified with

823 subjects total. Tramadol appeared to be generally beneficial and had a relatively low side effect profile over the short duration of these studies.

Unfortunately, only 2 studies were double-blind. Two were single blind crossover studies and the last was a single blind non—placebo-controlled study. Four of the 5 studies enrolled 64 patients or fewer; indeed, a single study by Bar-Or accounts for 604 (73%) of the total pool of patients. Furthermore, there was some heterogeneity in the definition of PE used, and it is not clear from the report how many men in each study had primary (lifelong) PE versus secondary (acquired) PE. As primary and secondary PE are thought to be different conditions with respect to etiology and treatment it is perhaps inadvisable to pool data from all 823 patients.

Given the heterogeneity of the data the authors wisely did not perform a meta-analysis; that said, it is something of a misnomer to characterize this manuscript as a systematic review as meta-analysis is the fundamental statistical core of systematic reviews. We must conclude from this that tramadol may have utility but more robust and better designed studies are required to determine when and where it should be used for treatment of PE.

A. W. Shindel, MD

Intratunical Injection of Human Adipose Tissue—derived Stem Cells Prevents Fibrosis and Is Associated with Improved Erectile Function in a Rat Model of Peyronie's Disease

Castiglione F, Hedlund P, Van der Aa F, et al (Univ Vita-Salute San Raffaele, Milan, Italy; Univ of Leuven, Belgium; et al)
Eur Urol 63:551-560, 2013

Background.—Peyronie's disease (PD) is a connective tissue disorder of the tunica albuginea (TA). Currently, no gold standard has been developed for the treatment of the disease in its active phase.

Objective.—To test the effects of a local injection of adipose tissue—derived stem cells (ADSCs) in the active phase of a rat model of PD on the subsequent development of fibrosis and elastosis of the TA and underlying erectile tissue.

Design, Setting, and Participants.—A total of 27 male 12-wk-old Sprague-Dawley rats were divided in three equal groups and underwent injection of vehicle (sham), 50-μg transforming growth factor (TGF)-β1 in a 50-μl vehicle in either a PD or a PD plus ADSC group in the dorsal aspect of the TA.

Intervention.—The sham and PD groups were treated 1 d after TGF-β1 injection with intralesional treatment of vehicle, and the PD plus ADSC group received 1 million human-labeled ADSCs in the 50-μl vehicle. Five weeks after treatment, six rats per group underwent erectile function measurement. Following euthanasia, penises were harvested for histology and Western blot.

Outcome Measurements and Statistical Analysis.—The ratio of intracavernous pressure to mean arterial pressure (ICP/MAP) upon cavernous nerve stimulation, elastin, and collagen III protein expression and histo-morphometric analysis of the penis. Statistical analysis was performed by analysis of variance followed by the Tukey-Kramer test for post hoc comparisons or the Mann-Whitney test when applicable.

Results and Limitations.—Erectile function significantly improved after ADSC treatment (ICP/MAP 0.37 in PD vs 0.59 in PD plus ADSC at 5-V stimulation; $p = 0.03$). PD animals developed areas of fibrosis and elastosis with a significant upregulation of collagen III and elastin protein expression. These fibrotic changes were prevented by ADSC treatment.

Conclusions.—This study is the first to test stem cell therapy in an animal model of PD. Injection of ADSCs into the TA during the active phase of PD prevents the formation of fibrosis and elastosis in the TA and corpus cavernosum.

▶ This article expands the ever-growing list of conditions potentially amenable to stem cell therapies to include Peyronie disease (PD). The current absence of any widely approved therapy for PD and the accessible location of the penis make this an ideal target for further development.

These authors report that stem cell treatment minimized tissue changes (eg, collagen deposition, buildup of disorganized elastin plaques) associated with injection of transforming growth factor beta (TGF-β) into the penis of Sprague-Dawley rats. Furthermore, stem cell therapy enhanced erectile response as assessed by intracavernous pressure measurement during cavernous nerve electrostimulation.

The injection of stem cells occurred one day post-injection of TGF-β. Whether this timing is reflective of the typical timing of presentation for treatment in men with PD is an open question. The TGF-β model itself may not be perfectly reflective of PD in humans, but it does represent the best available means for assessment at the current time.

It is important to note that the authors of this study used human-derived stem cells from a female subject. This cross-species stem cell transfer is interesting but will obviously not be suitable for future therapies; patients are very likely to prefer their own stem cells. Fortunately (perhaps), adipose tissue is quite plentiful worldwide, particularly in developed nations; it seems likely that stem cell reservoirs will be more than adequate for future needs should adipose-derived stem cells emerge as a leading therapy in the future.

We will eagerly await further developments in stem cell therapy in general and stem cells for PD in particular.

A. W. Shindel, MD

Prostate cancer diagnosis is associated with an increased risk of erectile dysfunction after prostate biopsy
Helfand BT, Glaser AP, Rimar K, et al (Northwestern Univ, Chicago, IL)
BJU Int 111:38-43, 2013

Objective.—• To evaluate prospectively the characteristics, erectile function and lower urinary tract symptoms (LUTS) of men undergoing prostate needle biopsy (PNBx).

Patients and Methods.—• From 2008 to 2011, 134 men were prospectively administered the International Index of Erectile Function (IIEF), American Urological Association Symptom Index (AUA-SI), and quality-of-life (QoL) questionnaires before and after undergoing a single 12-core PNBx.

• Comparisons of IIEF and AUA-SI scores before and after PNBx, based upon baseline characteristics and prostate cancer (PCa) diagnosis, were performed.

• Univariable and multivariable logistic regression models were used to characterize predictors of change in IIEF scores.

Results.—• In the 85 men who fulfilled the inclusion criteria, there were no significant differences between the mean (SD) total pre-biopsy and the mean (SD) post-biopsy IIEF scores: 57.8 (12.9) vs 54.3 (17.2).

• Subgroup analysis showed that men who had biopsy-proven PCa had significantly greater changes in their post-biopsy IIEF scores compared with men without (−10.1 vs. 1.0; $P < 0.001$).

• After specific analyses of the IIEF domains in these groups we found significant decreases in every domain, including erectile function ($P = 0.01$). On multivariate analyses, only PCa diagnosis was associated with a significant change in IIEF (odds ratio 7.2; $P = 0.003$).

• There were no differences in AUA-SI or QoL scores in the overall population or in subgroups.

Conclusions.—• Cancer diagnosis appears to have an adverse effect on the erectile function of men undergoing PNBx but no effect on LUTS. This study highlights a potential negative psychological confounder that may influence erectile function before the treatment of PCa.

• Additional prospective trials evaluating these relationships are warranted.

▶ Means for accurate assessment of erectile function before, during, and after radical prostatectomy has been a concern since the anatomic radical prostatectomy with nerve sparing was introduced. Casual questioning by the operating surgeon on pre- and postsurgery erectile function has been supplanted with validated measures and objective questionnaires designed to capture subtle nuances of impaired sexual function, which may occur after radical prostatectomy. These new measures are certainly improvements but do carry their own limitations.

A particular limitation is that "preprocedure" erectile function is often assessed shortly after the prostate cancer diagnosis is given. It is natural to assume that a majority of men experience marked changes in their sexual feelings and functionality after being given a cancer diagnosis. When later asked to characterize their sexual function before diagnosis/procedure, it is only human and entirely natural that many men will mischaracterize their erectile functionality, consciously or not.

This difficulty in characterizing erectile function is a fundamental challenge in accurate measurement and study of erectile function recovery after prostate cancer diagnosis/treatment. This interesting study demonstrates that prostate cancer diagnosis is clearly and independently associated with a decline in erectile function after prostate biopsy. This is hardly surprising and does not revolutionize clinical management. However, it is something that researchers who study sexual recovery after prostate cancer treatment should keep in mind. The precise timing of "baseline" erectile function assessment is obviously of critical import and should be detailed in future studies.

A. W. Shindel, MD

The Effect of Endovascular Revascularization of Common Iliac Artery Occlusions on Erectile Function
Gur S, Ozkan U, Onder H, et al (Sifa Hosp, Basmane, Izmir, Turkey; Baskent Univ, Yüregir, Adana, Turkey; Dicle Univ, Diyarbakir, Turkey)
Cardiovasc Intervent Radiol 36:84-89, 2013

Purpose.—To determine the incidence of erectile dysfunction in patients with common iliac artery (CIA) occlusive disease and the effect of revascularization on erectile function using the sexual health inventory for males (SHIM) questionnaire.

Methods.—All patients (35 men; mean age 57 ± 5 years; range 42–67 years) were asked to recall their sexual function before and 1 month after iliac recanalization. Univariate and multivariate analyses were performed to determine variables effecting improvement of impotence.

Results.—The incidence of impotence in patients with CIA occlusion was 74% (26 of 35) preoperatively. Overall 16 (46%) of 35 patients reported improved erectile function after iliac recanalization. The rate of improvement of impotence was 61.5% (16 of 26 impotent patients). Sixteen patients (46%), including seven with normal erectile function before the procedure, had no change. Three patients (8%) reported deterioration of their sexual function, two of whom (6%) had normal erectile function before the procedure. The median SHIM score increased from 14 (range 4–25) before the procedure to 20 (range 1–25) after the procedure ($P = 0.005$). The type of recanalization, the age of the patients, and the length of occlusion were related to erectile function improvement in univariate analysis. However, these factors were not independent factors for improvement of erectile dysfunction in multivariate analysis ($P > 0.05$).

Conclusion.—Endovascular recanalization of CIA occlusions clearly improves sexual function. More than half of the patients with erectile dysfunction who underwent endovascular recanalization of the CIA experienced improvement.

▶ The authors of this article report on recovery of erectile function after restoration of blood flow in the common iliac artery by revascularization using endovascular stents. Follow-up time points ranged from 1 to 6 months postprocedure.

In patients with erectile dysfunction (ED) at baseline, a slight majority (61%) reported improvement in erectile function. In the results section, the authors report that recovery was complete, satisfactory, and moderate in 6, 9, and 1 patients, respectively, although they do not clearly define what these terms mean in this context. However, 3 men reported a decline, including 2 who had been potent before the procedure.

This study is hampered by short-term follow-up and somewhat limited characterization of sexual function and activity before and after the treatment. It is an interesting concept and may have utility in the management of ED in the future; it has been suggested that prepenile circulation including the iliac and its pudendal branch are significant contributors to penile vascular-resistant and impaired-penile blood flow.[1] More robust studies with detailed end points including penile Doppler ultrasound assessment are warranted. Until such data are available, endovascular stenting for ED must be regarded as experimental.

A. W. Shindel, MD

Reference

1. Hannan JL, Blaser MC, Oldfield L, et al. Morphological and functional evidence for the contribution of the pudendal artery in aging-induced erectile dysfunction. *J Sex Med.* 2010;7:3373-3384.

Outcome of Penile Revascularization for Arteriogenic Erectile Dysfunction After Pelvic Fracture Urethral Injuries
Zuckerman JM, McCammon KA, Tisdale BE, et al (Eastern Virginia Med School, Norfolk)
Urology 80:1369-1374, 2012

Objective.—To review our experience with penile revascularization for patients with bilateral occlusion of the deep internal pudendal arteries after pelvic fracture urethral injury (PFUI).

Materials and Methods.—We identified 17 patients who had undergone penile revascularization with end-to-side anastomosis of the deep inferior epigastric artery to the dorsal penile artery from July 1991 to December 2010. Success was defined as achieving erections sufficient for intercourse with or without pharmacologic assistance.

Results.—All patients had had a PFUI causing arterial insufficiency and erectile dysfunction not responsive to pharmacologic intervention. Of the 17 patients, 4 (24%) underwent revascularization before and 13 (76%) after PFUI repair. The mean age at revascularization was 32.7 years (range

17-54). At an average follow-up of 3.1 years, the surgery was successful in 14 of the 17 patients (82%). In patients with erectile dysfunction as an indication for surgery, successful erections were achieved in 11 of 13. For those who underwent revascularization to prevent ischemic stenosis of the urethral repair, 3 of 4 achieved successful erections, and all subsequent urethral surgeries were successful. The penile duplex ultrasound parameters showed clinically and statistically significant improvements after revascularization. No operative complications developed. The average hospital length of stay was 4.7 days. Four patients experienced early postoperative complications, including an abdominal wall hematoma requiring evacuation in one, penile edema in two, and a superficial surgical site infection in one. No late complications occurred.

Conclusion.—Penile arterial revascularization in select patients can allow for successful treatment of PFUIs and the refractory erectile dysfunction caused by them.

▶ Penile revascularization is a specialized technique for management of erectile dysfunction (ED) in young healthy men who have suffered vascular trauma. It remains somewhat controversial given a dearth of large-scale reports on efficacy, but it should be considered in select cases because it is one of the few medical interventions that can actually lead to cure of ED.

This retrospective report from the practice of a leading expert in revascularization and reconstructive surgery of the penis indicates good functional outcomes in a small group of 17 young men with trauma-related ED. By and large, objective and subjective parameters improved in the treatment groups and the adverse event profile was favorable. All but one of the treatment successes (n = 14) remained reliant on some form of erectogenic therapy. The follow-up for this cohort was somewhat heterogeneous, with a fair number of patients not seen again in the author's practice but rather returned to their primary referring urologist.

In the end, penile revascularization will likely remain a footnote in the armamentarium of ED treatment options, but it may be a very important footnote for appropriately selected patients.

A. W. Shindel, MD

Priapism is Associated with Sleep Hypoxemia in Sickle Cell Disease
Roizenblatt M, Figueiredo MS, Cançado RD, et al (Universidade Federal de Sao Paulo, Brazil; et al)
J Urol 188:1245-1251, 2012

Purpose.—We assessed penile rigidity during sleep and the relationship of sleep abnormalities with priapism in adults with sickle cell disease.

Materials and Methods.—This was a case-control study of 18 patients with sickle cell disease and a history of priapism during the previous year, and 16 controls with sickle cell disease. Participants underwent overnight polysomnography and RigiScan® Plus recording to detect penile rigidity oscillations.

Results.—The priapism group (cases) showed a higher apnea-hypopnea index and oxyhemoglobin desaturation parameters than controls. A lower positive correlation between the apnea-hypopnea index and oxyhemoglobin desaturation time was observed in cases than in controls (Spearman coefficient $\rho = 0.49$, $p = 0.05$ vs $\rho = 0.76$, $p < 0.01$), suggesting that desaturation events occurred independently of apnea. Two controls and 14 cases had a total sleep time that was greater than 10% with oxyhemoglobin saturation less than 90% but without CO_2 retention. Penile rigidity events were observed during rapid eye movement sleep and during stage 2 of nonrapid eye movement sleep, particularly in cases. The duration of penile rigidity events concomitant to respiratory events was higher in cases than in controls. Regression analysis revealed that the periodic limb movement and desaturation indexes were associated with priapism after adjusting for rapid eye movement sleep and lung involvement. Finally, oxyhemoglobin saturation less than 90% was associated with priapism after adjusting for lung involvement, hyperhemolysis and the apnea-hypopnea index.

Conclusions.—Oxyhemoglobin desaturation during sleep was associated with priapism history. It may underlie the distribution pattern of penile rigidity events during sleep in these patients.

▶ Priapism attracts relatively little attention and so any publications on this vexing condition are a welcome addition to our knowledge base. This case-control study investigates 2 populations of sickle cell patients, one with priapism history (cases) and another without (controls). It is concluded that blood oxygen desaturation was more pronounced in the cases; this was associated with apnea and other breathing parameters. RigiScan measurements were used as a proxy for erectile tumescence. It is unclear what to make of these data, at least in the sense of what to do clinically. However, this finding opens the door for more investigations; perhaps improvement of oxygenation during sleep can reduce priapism episodes? Will assessment by sleep specialists and/or pulmonologists contribute to management of patients with sickle cell-associated priapism? Given the generally poor understanding of sickle cell disease—associated priapism, these data are a welcome addition indeed. We will eagerly await the next round of findings.

A. W. Shindel, MD

The Impact of Serial Prostate Biopsies on Sexual Function in Men on Active Surveillance for Prostate Cancer
Hilton JF, Blaschko SD, Whitson JM, et al (Univ of California-San Francisco)
J Urol 188:1252-1259, 2012

Purpose.—NCCN Guidelines® recommend annual prostate biopsies for men with low risk prostate cancer on active surveillance. We determined whether erectile function decreases with the number of biopsies experienced.

Materials and Methods.—During a median 3.2-year followup after prostate cancer diagnosis in 2003 to 2010 at our institution 427 men on active surveillance underwent a total of 1,197 biopsies and provided 1,398 erectile function evaluations via the Sexual Health Inventory for Men questionnaire. For analysis we decomposed the 25-point questionnaire responses into a 5-point erectile function score and a 3-level sexual activity status. We used separate models adjusted for patient characteristics to determine whether either outcome varied with biopsy exposure.

Results.—At diagnosis the median age was 61 years and median prostate specific antigen was 5.3 ng/ml. Of the cases 70% were clinical stage cT1 and 93% were Gleason score less than 7. Of biopsies followed by evaluations 40% were the first undergone by the patient and 9% were the fifth to ninth. At the first erectile function evaluation 15% of men were inactive, 8% engage in stimulation and 77% engaged in intercourse. Sexual activity level changed in greater than 20% of respondents between evaluations. Adjusted erectile function scores were not associated with biopsy exposure cross-sectionally or longitudinally but they corresponded with the 50th, 63rd and 80th percentiles of erectile function by increasing sexual activity level. Similarly, sexual activity was not associated with biopsy exposure. Separated outcomes were more accurate and informative than Sexual Health Inventory for Men scores.

Conclusions.—Our study had high power to detect erectile function-biopsy associations but it estimated that the effects were negligible. We recommend erectile function scores over Sexual Health Inventory for Men scores to avoid biased assessment of erectile function.

► The authors of this study report that there is no evidence in their institutional series that prostate biopsy is associated with increased rates of erectile dysfunction (ED) in a cohort of men undergoing active surveillance for prostate cancer. The authors utilized the Sexual Health Inventory for Men (SHIM) but subjected it to some interesting modifications, specifically dividing the total SHIM score by the number of questions answered to produce a continuous value between 1 and 5. The authors justify this by citing a high degree of correlation between individual SHIM components. Be that as it may, it's unclear to me whether this manipulation leaves the validity of this instrument intact. I would answer "no." To their credit, the authors do report SHIM scores within the text; while there appears to be a decline in mean SHIM score, this decline is of unclear significance as a mean; it would be interesting to know the characteristics of the men who did experience a clinically relevant (approximately 4 point) decline in SHIM score after biopsy.

Another limitation is that the authors did not assess sexual activity but rather extrapolated this from SHIM scores and assumed that those with scores of 1–5 were inactive patients and those with scores of 6–10 were patients who engaged in stimulation only—presumably masturbation without penetration. It is not necessarily accurate to assume sexual activity based on the SHIM score alone, particularly in light of the aforementioned modifications to the SHIM itself.

This complex analysis using a reductionist approach to an instrument intended and validated as a 5-item instrument makes me very uneasy about casual acceptance of these data as proof of the benignity of repeat prostate biopsy. Of course, this is not evidence of a negative effect either; the change in SHIM score was (on average) not clearly statistically significant. More research is needed.

A. W. Shindel, MD

Avanafil for the Treatment of Erectile Dysfunction: A Multicenter, Randomized, Double-Blind Study in Men With Diabetes Mellitus

Goldstein I, Jones LA, Belkoff LH, et al (Alvarado Hosp, San Diego, CA; Urology San Antonio Res, TX; Urologic Consultants of Southeastern Pennsylvania, Bala Cynwyd; et al)

Mayo Clin Proc 87:843-852, 2012

Objective.—To prospectively assess the safety and effectiveness of the investigational phosphodiesterase 5 inhibitor avanafil to treat erectile dysfunction in men with diabetes mellitus.

Patients and Methods.—This 12-week, multicenter, double-blind, placebo-controlled study conducted between December 15, 2008, and February 11, 2010, randomized 390 men with diabetes and erectile dysfunction 1:1:1 to receive avanafil, 100 mg (n = 129), avanafil, 200 mg (n = 131), or placebo (n = 130). Coprimary end points assessed changes in the percentage of sexual attempts in which men were able to maintain an erection of sufficient duration to have successful intercourse (Sexual Encounter Profile [SEP] 3), percentage of sexual attempts in which men were able to insert the penis into the partner's vagina (SEP 2), and International Index of Erectile Function erectile function domain score.

Results.—Compared with placebo, least-squares mean change from baseline to study end in SEP 3, SEP 2, and International Index of Erectile Function erectile function domain score were significantly improved with both avanafil, 100 mg ($P \leq .002$), and avanafil, 200 mg ($P < .001$). Additional analyses indicated that successful intercourse could be initiated in 15 minutes or less through more than 6 hours after avanafil dosing. Adverse events most commonly reported with avanafil treatment were headache, nasopharyngitis, flushing, and sinus congestion.

Conclusion.—Avanafil was safe and effective for treating erectile dysfunction in men with diabetes and was effective as early as 15 minutes and more than 6 hours after dosing. The adverse events seen with avanafil were similar to those seen with other phosphodiesterase 5 inhibitors.

Trial Registration.—clinicaltrials.gov Identifier NCT00809471.

▶ This randomized, controlled trial comes out in support of a new phosphodiesterase-5 inhibitor (PDE5I), avanafil. This drug was approved by the US Food and Drug Administration in the spring of 2012; as of this writing, it is not yet clinically available. The efficacy of avanafil in enhancing penile erections in this population of men with erectile dysfunction (ED) was significantly superior to that of placebo, and the side-effect profile was grossly similar to what is observed with other PDE5Is. Avanafil is an aminoheterocycle compound and thus has a markedly different chemical structure from sildenafil, vardenafil (both are pyrazolopyrimidines), and tadalafil. Whether this will fundamentally represent a change, let alone improvement, in clinical efficacy for the PDE5I class is at this time unclear. Certainly, there is little detriment to having an additional oral PDE5I available, and it is very likely that some American men may wind up preferring this medication compared with any of the other three. That said, we are still waiting (somewhat patiently) for the next paradigm-shifting ED drug, one that will target an enzyme or process other than PDE5.

A. W. Shindel, MD

Effect of Tunical Defect Size After Peyronie's Plaque Excision on Postoperative Erectile Function: Do Centimeters Matter?

Kozacioglu Z, Degirmenci T, Gunlusoy B, et al (Bozyaka Training and Res Hosp Urology Clinic Izmir, Turkey)
Urology 80:1051-1055, 2012

Objective.—To demonstrate the effect of the size of the resultant tunical defect after plaque excision on postoperative erectile function of patients with Peyronie's disease.

Methods.—The results of 38 patients with plaque excision and dermal grafting were reviewed from April 2007 to June 2011. History, physical examination, self-shot photograph, color duplex ultrasonography were done preoperatively, and the risk factors for erectile dysfunction were evaluated. The tunical defects were ≥ 3 cm for group 1 and < 3 cm for group 2. The postoperative need for phosphodiesterase type 5 inhibitors was noted for both groups. The International Index of Erectile Function-5 questionnaire was completed by all patients.

Results.—Overall, phosphodiesterase type 5 inhibitors were necessary for 13 (34%) of 38 patients; 7 (58.3%) of 12 in group 1 and 6 (23%) of 26 in group 2. The risk factors for postoperative erectile dysfunction were statistically similar for both groups. If patients with ventral defects were excluded from group 2, the number of patients requiring phosphodiesterase type 5 inhibitors was 4 (17%) of 24. The patients in group 2 answered the fifth question (4.6 ± 0.55) significantly different from those in group 1 (3.7 ± 0.88).

Conclusion.—Plaque excision and dermal grafting can be recommended only for highly selected patients with Peyronie's disease with good erectile capacity, with a degree of angle not suitable for only plication or Nesbit techniques, for patients who do not accept any significant shortening of the penis, and if the size of the tunical defect will be < 3 cm. Additional techniques on the opposite aspect of the lesion are advocated for the remaining curvatures, not to enlarge the tunical defect > 3 cm.

▶ This article reports that defect size is an important predictor of new onset erectile dysfunction (ED) and PDE5I reliance after tunical excision and dermal grafting for Peyronie's disease.

The authors present data indicating that none of the other comorbid factors assessed (tobacco use, hypertension, diabetes) were not significant. While somewhat reassuring, it is unfortunate that the list of comorbid factors assessed seems so limited and that a multivariate analysis was not conducted to verify the independent influence of tunica defect size. One might also wonder whether some other variable that led to need for larger excision defect at surgery is responsible for the observed results. It is also unclear that the authors selected the ideal cutoff for significance of defect size; they report that they simply checked differences in 0.25-cm intervals until they reached a level of significance. This is hardly the best way to establish cutoffs.

It's hard to argue that larger defects are better, but this study could have been better designed to set optimal parameters.

A. W. Shindel, MD

Pilot Genome-Wide Association Search Identifies Potential Loci for Risk of Erectile Dysfunction in Type 1 Diabetes Using the DCCT/EDIC Study Cohort
Hotaling JM, the DCCT/EDIC Research Group (Univ of Washington School of Medicine, Seattle; et al)
J Urol 188:514-520, 2012

Purpose.—We identified genetic predictors of diabetes associated erectile dysfunction using genome-wide and candidate gene approaches in a cohort of men with type 1 diabetes.

Materials and Methods.—We examined 528 white men with type 1 diabetes, including 125 with erectile dysfunction, from DCCT (Diabetes Control and Complications Trial) and its observational followup, the EDIC (Epidemiology of Diabetes Interventions and Complications) study. Erectile dysfunction was identified from a single International Index of Erectile Function item. A Human1M BeadChip (Illumina®) was used for genotyping. A total of 867,125 single nucleotide polymorphisms were subjected to analysis. Whole genome and candidate gene approaches were used to test the hypothesis that genetic polymorphisms may predispose men with type 1 diabetes to erectile dysfunction. Univariate and multivariate models were used, controlling for age, HbA1c, diabetes duration and prior randomization to intensive or conventional insulin therapy during DCCT. A stratified false discovery rate was used to perform the candidate gene approach.

Results.—Two single nucleotide polymorphisms located on chromosome 3 in 1 genomic loci were associated with erectile dysfunction with

$p < 1 \times 10^{-6}$, including rs9810233 with $p = 7 \times 10^{-7}$ and rs1920201 with $p = 9 \times 10^{-7}$. The nearest gene to these 2 single nucleotide polymorphisms is ALCAM. Genetic association results at these loci were similar on univariate and multivariate analysis. No candidate genes met the criteria for statistical significance.

Conclusions.—Two single nucleotide polymorphisms, rs9810233 and rs1920101, which are 25 kb apart, are associated with erectile dysfunction, although they do not meet the standard genome-wide association study significance criterion of $p < 5 \times 10^{-8}$. Other studies with larger sample sizes are required to determine whether ALCAM represents a novel gene in the pathogenesis of diabetes associated erectile dysfunction.

▶ The genome and epigenome have emerged as a new frontier for investigation and study of risk factors for erectile dysfunction (ED). In this study, a population of white men with diabetes was studied using whole genome assays to identify polymorphisms that were more prevalent in the men with diagnosed ED (in this study, men who reported low or very low on a single question of the IIEF pertaining to confidence attaining and maintaining erection).

Two single nucleotide polymorphisms with higher prevalence in men with ED were identified on chromosome 3, nearest to a gene that produces a protein that modulates leukocyte adhesion. Based on the sheer volume of data analyzed in a study such as this, very strict criteria for statistical significance must be selected, as the possibility of type I error is very high with so many tests being run. This strict criterion (*P* < .00000005) was not met for these 2 single nucleotide polymorphisms; whether this is a statistical limitation or represents a genuine absence of difference is unclear. It is also not entirely clear how a gene that likely modulates leukocyte activity is related to ED, although mechanisms such as oxidative stress and inflammation may play a role.

Regardless, this is exciting technology that holds the promise of personalized medicine. Additional studies are warranted in white and nonwhite populations.

A. W. Shindel, MD

Efficacy and Safety of Tramadol for Premature Ejaculation: A Systematic Review and Meta-analysis
Wu T, Yue X, Duan X, et al (Sichuan Univ, Chengdu, China)
Urology 80:618-624, 2012

Objective.—To present a systematic review to assess efficacy and safety of tramadol for premature ejaculation.

Methods.—A literature search was performed using the Cochrane Library, MEDLINE, EMBASE, and Science Citation Index Expanded. Literature reviewed included meta-analyses and randomized and nonrandomized prospective studies. End points included intravaginal ejaculation latency time (in minutes), adverse events, and patient-reported outcome assessments. We used mean difference to measure intravaginal ejaculation latency time and odds ratio to measure adverse events rates. These odds ratios were pooled using a random or fixed effects model and were tested for heterogeneity. We used the Cochrane Collaboration's Review manager (RevMan) 5.1 software for statistical analysis.

Results.—We identified 7 publications that strictly met our eligibility criteria. Meta-analysis of extractable data showed that tramadol was associated with a 3-minute intravaginal ejaculation latency time increasing (mean difference 2.77 minutes; 95% CI 1.12-4.47; $P = .001$) and significantly more patients with adverse events rates compared with placebo (odds ratio 2.89; 95% CI 1.88-4.43; $P < .0001$). There were no differences between the tramadol and the paroxetine of intravaginal ejaculation latency time (mean difference -0.44; 95% CI -5.07 to 4.18; $P = .85$). In addition, patients saw significantly greater improvement in patient-reported outcome.

Conclusion.—In this diverse population, tramadol is an effective and safety pharmacologic therapy for premature ejaculation.

▶ Tramadol has attracted some attention as a means to treat premature ejaculation (PE). In the absence of any US Food and Drug Administration—approved therapy, an addition to the pharmaceutical armamentarium would be quite welcome. This meta-analysis reports that tramadol as an on-demand therapy is significantly superior to placebo for management of PE at the expense of markedly more adverse events (particularly somnolence and gastrointestinal upset) compared with placebo. There appeared to be general equivalence of efficacy between tramadol and the off-label oral therapy for PE that is most commonly prescribed. Unfortunately, the trials that were included exhibited some heterogeneity so it's hard to know how this drug would be best prescribed for premature ejaculation. Whether tramadol will have a role in PE is unclear; there is some concern that this drug may carry the potential for addiction. Larger studies with more rigorous criteria for enrollment and outcome are required to clearly define the role of tramadol in management of ejaculation disorders.

A. W. Shindel, MD

Coated Implants and "No Touch" Surgical Technique Decreases Risk of Infection in Inflatable Penile Prosthesis Implantation to 0.46%
Eid JF, Wilson SK, Cleves M, et al (Advanced Urologic Care, NY; Inst for Urologic Excellence, Indio, CA; UAMS, Little Rock, AR; et al)
Urology 79:1310-1316, 2012

Objective.—To explore whether a "no touch" enhancement to the surgical technique of inflatable penile prosthesis (IPPs) implantaion will further decrease infection rates.

Materials and Methods.—A single surgeon performed 2347 IPPs between January 2002 and June 2011. Patients receiving each manufacturer's implants were stratified for age and diabetes. Since 2003, infection retardant—coated IPPs were implanted through the standardized penoscrotal approach. Since 2006, the "no touch" enhancement was added to the surgical procedure. Infection rates in the noncoated IPP, coated IPP with standard technique, and coated IPP implanted with "no touch" enhancement were calculated and subjected to statistical analysis. The two company's implants were scrutinized for their individual infection rates in each group.

Results.—Patients in all the groups were similar for age and diabetes. 132 noncoated implants had an infection rate of 5.3%. In the years 2003-2005, 704 coated devices had a statistically significant improvement in incidence of infection to 2%. In the years 2006-2010, the "no touch" technique enhanced the standard surgical procedure in 1511 patients. Only 7 infections were seen yielding an infection incidence of 0.46%. There was no difference in the two manufacturer's infection rates. Differentiation between virgin and revision operation displayed no bias in the infection rate.

Conclusion.—Infection-retardant coatings lower the risk of infection from 5.3% to 2%. The "no touch" enhancement to the surgical procedure further decreases the rate of infection to 0.46%. Neither manufacturer showed statistical superiority in survival from revision for infection.

▶ The authors of this article are among the most famous penile implant surgeons in practice today. In the experienced hands of this authorial team, it is reported that there was marked decline in penile implant infection rates after introduction of implant cylinders coated with antibiotics or with a hydrophilic compound that permits absorption followed by slow elution of an antibiotic of choice. It is rare to see noncoated implants in use these days; the modification that may, however, be less utilized but worthy of consideration by penile prosthesis surgeons is the no-touch technique of Eid, which was associated with a further decline in infection rate after adoption. These are clearly associations only, but the temporal relationship certainly suggests that coating and no-touch make a big difference in infection rates. These interventions are generally straightforward and should not pose prohibitive difficulty for most surgeons, although placement of the second no-touch drape will likely add some time early on in its adoption. It is also unclear how this approach could be adapted for infrapubic dissections. It must be emphasized that these data represent results from some of the most experienced prosthetic surgeons in the world. Other penile implant surgeons should aspire to this level of mastery; however, it would be prudent when speaking to patients to quote one's own rate of infection and other complications rather than the results of acknowledged leaders in the field.

A. W. Shindel, MD

Erectile Function, Incontinence, and Other Quality of Life Outcomes Following Proton Therapy for Prostate Cancer in Men 60 Years Old and Younger

Hoppe BS, Nichols RC, Henderson RH, et al (Univ of Florida Proton Therapy Inst, Jacksonville; et al)
Cancer 118:4619-4626, 2012

Background.—This study sought to evaluate patient-reported health-related quality of life following proton therapy for prostate cancer in men ≤ 60 years old.

Methods.—Between August 2006 and January 2010, 262 hormone-naive men ≤ 60 years old were treated with definitive proton therapy for prostate cancer. Before treatment and every 6 months after treatment, patients filled out the Expanded Prostate Index Composite (EPIC) and the International Index of Erectile Function (IIEF) questionnaires. Potency was defined as successful sexual intercourse in the prior month or an EPIC sexual summary (SS) score ≥ 60.

Results.—Median follow-up was 24 months; 90% of men completed follow-up EPIC forms within the last year. For EPIC urinary, bowel, and hormone subscales, the average decline from baseline to 2 years was ≤ 5 points, except for bowel function (5.2 points). SS scores declined 12.6 points after 2 years. Potency rates declined by 11% from baseline at 2 years, but 94% of men were potent with a baseline IIEF > 21, body mass index < 30, and no history of diabetes. At 2 years after treatment, only 1.8% of men required a pad for urge incontinence. On multivariate analysis, factors associated with a significant decline in SS score were mean penile bulb dose ≥ 40 cobalt Gy equivalents ($P = .012$) and radiation dose ≥ 80 cobalt Gy equivalents ($P = .017$); only diabetes was significantly associated with impotence ($P = .015$).

Conclusions.—Young men undergoing proton therapy for treatment of prostate cancer have excellent outcomes with respect to erectile dysfunction, urinary incontinence, and other health-related quality of life parameters during the first 2 years after treatment. Longer follow-up is needed to confirm these findings.

▶ The authors of this study report on urinary, bowel, and sexual function after treatment of prostate cancer with proton beam as monotherapy. They conclude that proton beam therapy has generally favorable outcomes with respect to sexual function as assessed by the Expanded Prostate Index Composite (EPIC). Indeed, nonobese men without diabetes and good erectile function at baseline had a 94% potency rate (defined below) at 2 years.

The definition of sexual potency (EPIC score > 60 or successful intercourse in the past month) is somewhat suboptimal in that success is subjective. Use of the more descriptive Sexual Encounter Profile Questions 2 and 3 would have been more informative and reliable.

It is important to note that EPIC sexual function composite score and the International Index of Erectile Function (IIEF)-EF total score declined significantly over the period of the study. Some of this is to be expected by natural aging, but it is indubitably the case that proton beam therapy can only exert deleterious effects on erectile function, so it is parsimonious to conclude that this therapy does carry some risk of worsening ED. That said, the sexual function side-effect profile in this population of men younger than 60 is generally acceptable and suggests that this may be an acceptable treatment modality for some men undergoing definitive therapy for prostate cancer.

A. W. Shindel, MD

Efficacy and Safety of Udenafil for Erectile Dysfunction: A Meta-analysis of Randomized Controlled Trials

Ding H, Du W, Wang H et al (Second Hosp of Lanzhou Univ, China; Med College of Shandong Univ, Jinan City, China; et al)
Urology 80:134-139, 2012

Objective.—To systematically review the evidence on the efficacy and safety of udenafil as treatment of erectile dysfunction from randomized controlled trials.

Methods.—We searched PubMed, Embase, and the Cochrane Library database up to October 2011. The outcome measures assessed were the change from baseline for the International Index of Erectile Function erectile function domain score (primary), the change from baseline for Sexual Encounter Profile questions 2 and 3, the shift to normal rate (erectile function domain ≥ 26), the response to the Global Assessment Questionnaire and adverse effects (secondary). Two of us independently assessed the study quality and extracted data. All data were analyzed using Review Manager, version 5.0.2.

Results.—Five randomized controlled trials totaling 1109 patients were included. At the follow-up endpoints, udenafil was found to be more effective than placebo, and the tolerability was good. The pooled results showed that the udenafil group was significantly greater than the placebo group in the change from baseline for the International Index of Erectile Function erectile function domain score (mean difference 5.65, 95% confidence interval 4.41-6.89, $P < .00001$). All included studies indicated that most adverse events were mild or moderate in severity, and no serious adverse events were reported during the study period. The most common drug-related adverse events were flushing and headache (udenafil vs placebo, 5.6% vs 1.8% and 3.1% vs 0%, respectively).

Conclusion.—The results from the current meta-analysis have suggested that udenafil is an effective and well-tolerated therapy for erectile dysfunction. The findings of the present review highlight the need for more efficient performance of higher quality, large-sample, various-race, long-term, randomized controlled trials to verify the efficacy and safety of udenafil.

▶ Udenafil is a PDE5 inhibitor medication available in several countries around the world (South Korea, Turkey, and others) but not currently available in the

United States. This meta-analysis highlights the efficacy profile of udenafil for management of erectile dysfunction (ED); it is clear that this medication is efficacious and has a favorable side-effect profile.

Currently, 4 PDE5 inhibitors are approved for use in the United States. Several other PDE5 inhibitors are either approved or at various stages of development around the world. These medications differ in their structures, side-effect profiles, dosing options, and pharmacokinetic profiles. Whether one is truly better than another is something of a moot point that will likely never be answered on a population level; the optimal medication for a given man will be whichever he personally prefers for whatever constellation of reasons. To that end, there is something to be gained by having a wide variety of options. However, it is my opinion that we will be better served by (1) developing new therapeutic targets for ED beyond inhibitors of PDE5 and (2) emphasizing prevention/reversal of ED by advocating healthier lifestyles.

A. W. Shindel, MD

Response to On-demand Vardenafil was Improved by its Daily Usage in Hypertensive Men

Javaroni V, Queiroz Miguez M, Burla A, et al (State Univ of Rio de Janeiro, Brazil)
Urology 80:858-864, 2012

Objective.—To evaluate whether the response to on-demand vardenafil could be improved by its daily usage in hypertensive men with erectile dysfunction (ED) who previously did not answer to on-demand regime.

Methods.—Our main efficacy criterion was per patient percentage of positive answers on the Sexual Encounter Profile question 3 (SEP3). Carotid intima-media thickness (IMT), flow-mediated dilation (FMD), and nitrate-mediated dilation on brachial artery were considered as vascular parameters. A total of 74 hypertensive men with ED aged 50 to 70 years with no major cardiovascular disease were selected from 284 patients initially referred. After vardenafil on-demand usage during 4 weeks, patients with more than 50% of positive answers on the SEP3, or 50% and more than 6 points on the International Index of Erectile Function-Erection Function Domain (IIEF-EF) basal score or positive answer to global evaluation question were considered "responders." "Nonresponders" (n = 35) were randomized to daily vardenafil 10 mg or placebo during 5 weeks along with open 10 mg of vardenafil before intercourse.

Results.—In the active group, 38.8% of patients became responders to vardenafil ($P < .05$). Clinical response to continuous vardenafil correlated with sexual frequency ($r = .68$, $P < .01$), Framingham risk score ($r = -.65$, $P < .01$), carotid IMT ($r = -.61$, $P = .01$) and low-density lipoprotein (LDL)-cholesterol ($r = -.64$, $P < .01$).

Conclusion.—Daily vardenafil during 5 weeks rescued response to on-demand regime among ED hypertensive men with no major cardiovascular disease. Further clinical trials and cost-effectiveness studies are necessary to confirm these findings.

▶ This interesting multiphase study examines the second stage of a vardenafil study; the population of men who did not experience at least a 50% rate of successful intercourse (maintenance of erection until orgasm) with vardenafil 20 mg on demand or a 6-point increase in the erectile function domain of the IIEF were randomly assigned to daily placebo versus vardenafil 10 mg with 10 mg of vardenafil open label on demand for intercourse.

The number of patients enrolled is quite small; it is implied based on the dosing regimens that the greater response in the daily vardenafil group was not mediated by higher doses; in the responder group for the second study, patients had previously not responded to 20 mg on demand but some responded with 10 mg on demand with 10 mg daily.

Better-designed studies have not convincingly established a benefit to daily dose of PDE5I for penile rehabilitation. While this study is interesting, it cannot by itself justify the potential expense of daily-dose vardenafil as a salvage therapy for PDE5I nonresponders.

A. W. Shindel, MD

Prevention and Management of Postprostatectomy Sexual Dysfunctions Part 1: Choosing the Right Patient at the Right Time for the Right Surgery
Salonia A, Burnett AL, Graefen M, et al (Univ Vita-Salute San Raffaele, Milan, Italy; The Johns Hopkins Hosp, Baltimore, MD; Univ Hamburg-Eppendorf, Germany; et al)
Eur Urol 62:261-272, 2012

Context.—Sexual dysfunction is common in patients following radical prostatectomy (RP) for prostate cancer (PCa).

Objective.—To review the available literature concerning prevention and management strategies for post-RP erectile function (EF) impairment in terms of preoperative patient characteristics and intra- and postoperative factors that may influence EF recovery.

Evidence acquisition.—A literature search was performed using Google and PubMed database for English-language original and review articles either published or e-published up to November 2011.

Evidence synthesis.—The literature demonstrates great inconsistency in what constitutes normal EF before surgery and what a man may consider a normal erection after RP. The use of validated psychometric instruments with recognised cut-offs for normalcy and severity during the pre- and post-operative evaluation should be routinely considered. Therefore, a comprehensive discussion with the patient about the true prevalence of postoperative erectile dysfunction (ED), the concept of spontaneous or pharmacologically assisted erections, and the difference between "back to baseline" EF and "erections adequate enough to have successful intercourse" clearly emerge as key issues in the eventual understanding of the prevention of ED and promotion of satisfactory EF recovery post-RP. Patient factors (including age, baseline EF, and status of comorbid conditions), cancer selection (unilateral vs bilateral nerve sparing), type of surgery (ie, intra- vs inter- vs extrafascial surgeries), surgical techniques (ie, open, laparoscopic, and robot-assisted RP), and surgeon factors (ie, surgical volume and surgical skill) represent the key significant contributors to EF recovery.

Conclusions.—The complexity of the issues discussed throughout this review culminates in the simple concept that optimal outcomes are achieved by the careful choice of the correct patient for the correct type of surgery.

▶ This excellent article is part of a series detailing the optimal management of sexual function in patients who are contemplating or have undergone radical prostatectomy for prostate malignancy. This article details the tremendous heterogeneity in reported outcomes and illustrates that much of this is caused by the wide variance in subject populations and definitions of what constitutes recovery of erectile function. It is stressed that very few patients maintain their baseline level of erectile rigidity postoperatively. A patient who has firm but not hard penile erection just sufficient to enable coitus when using an oral erectogenic therapy may be classified by researchers as potent; however, this man may not feel that he is adequately potent if before surgery he had a very hard, reliable erection with no need for oral therapy.

It is stressed here that realistic counseling about the degree and timing of erectile function recovery is essential. Counseling should also take into account patient and surgeon factors that influence the odds of erectile function recovery (nerve-sparing status, age, comorbidities, attention to vascular variability intraoperatively).

A. W. Shindel, MD

Population-based study of erectile dysfunction and polypharmacy
Londoño DC, Slezak JM, Quinn VP, et al (Kaiser Permanente Los Angeles Med Ctr, CA; Kaiser Permanente Southern California, Pasadena, CA; et al)
BJU Int 110:254-259, 2012

Objective.—To study the association between erectile dysfunction (ED) and polypharmacy use in a large, ethnically and racially diverse cohort of men enrolled in the California Men's Health Study (CMHS).

Patients and Methods.—Men from the Kaiser Permanente Southern California (KPSC) health plan, enrolled in the CMHS in 2002, had an age range of 45–69 years. ED and comorbidities of these subjects were identified by questionnaire responses.

The number of drugs taken was determined from the year before enrollment through electronic pharmacy records and questionnaire responses.

Results.—Among the 37 712 (KPSC) subjects, 10 717 (29%) reported moderate or severe ED.

Across all age groups, ED was more prevalent as the number of medications increased.

In men taking 0–2, 3–5,6–9 and $\geq$ 10 medications, the percentage of men reporting moderate ED was 15.9, 19.7, 25.5 and 30.9%, respectively ($P < 0.001$).

With adjustment for age, race, smoking, diabetes, hypertension, hyperlipidaemia, peripheral vascular disease, coronary artery disease and body mass index, men taking >10 drugs were more likely to have ED (odds ratio = 2.32, 95% confidence interval 2.14–2.52) with evidence of a dose-response relationship.

Conclusion.—These data suggest that the number of medications a man takes is associated with worse ED, even after comorbidities have been taken into account.

Study Typo.—Symptom prevalence (population cohort).

Level of Evidence.—1b.

What' s known on the subject? and What does the study add?

It is known that medical conditions such as diabetes, high blood pressure, high cholesterol, smoking and prescribed medications cause erectile dysfunction (ED). This has been studied at the molecular level and reported in population studies. The present study shows that, after accounting for known medical problems, there is a dose–response relationship, in which worsening degrees of ED are seen when a greater number of medications are taken, regardless if they are prescribed or over the counter.

The study can help primary care doctors and urologists to make a differential diagnosis of ED and it can also help improve patient's erectile function by tailoring and curtailing current medication use to maximize therapeutic benefit but minimize ED side effects in men, thus improving health-related quality of life.

▶ In this large population of men aged 45–69 from a managed care group, men using multiple medications were more likely to suffer from erectile dysfunction (ED). This relationship held even after adjustment for vascular and metabolic parameters that are known to be associated with higher prevalence of ED. This adjustment is obviously of critical import, as men who are taking many medicines will, as a rule, have more potential confounding comorbid conditions.

The authors used a definition of ED modified from the Massachusetts Male Aging Study that asked whether men can always, usually, sometimes, or never get an erection rigid enough for satisfactory intercourse. While not ideal, as a single-item patient-reported outcome this is a reasonable proxy measure for erectile capacity.

Whether it is within the scope of a urologist's practice to manage medication cessation is a separate issue; however, it can be deduced from this that when we are consulted for management of ED, one of our standard recommendations (in addition to encouraging healthy lifestyles and modification of reversible factors) should be medication cessation where feasible/safe. Particular attention should of course be devoted to cessation of medicines known to be risk factors for ED (eg, β-blockers, thiazides, antidepressants, hormone modulators).

A. W. Shindel, MD

The Princeton III Consensus Recommendations for the Management of Erectile Dysfunction and Cardiovascular Disease

Nehra A, Jackson G, Miner M, et al (Mayo Clinic, Rochester, MN; Guys and St Thomas Hosps London, UK; Brown Univ, Providence, RI; et al)
Mayo Clin Proc 87:766-778, 2012

The Princeton Consensus (Expert Panel) Conference is a multispecialty collaborative tradition dedicated to optimizing sexual function and preserving cardiovascular health. The third Princeton Consensus met November 8 to 10, 2010, and had 2 primary objectives. The first objective focused on the evaluation and management of cardiovascular risk in men with erectile dysfunction (ED) and no known cardiovascular disease (CVD), with particular emphasis on identification of men with ED who may require additional cardiologic work-up. The second objective focused on reevaluation and modification of previous recommendations for evaluation of cardiac risk associated with sexual activity in men with known CVD. The Panel's recommendations build on those developed during the first and second Princeton Consensus Conferences, first emphasizing the use of exercise ability and stress testing to ensure that each man's cardiovascular health is consistent with the physical demands of sexual activity before prescribing treatment for ED, and second highlighting the link between ED and CVD, which may be asymptomatic and may benefit from cardiovascular risk reduction.

▶ Now in its third iteration, the Princeton criteria supply the most up-to-date and evidence-based metrics by which to assess a patient's suitability for erectile dysfunction (ED) treatment. Beyond that, these data highlight the now well-established connections between cardiovascular disease and ED.

As a consensus statement, the Princeton III publication does not provide new data but rather summarizes existing recommendations. In general, this article highlights that erectile dysfunction is an independent risk factor for incidence cardiovascular disease, that men who have ED should be assessed for occult cardiac disease by a primary care physician or cardiologist, that modification of risk factors and/or treatment of occult vascular disease may alter progression to more serious cardiac disease and cardiac events, and that modification of disease factors should be instituted before treatment for ED is initiated in patients with high-risk cardiac disease (eg, refractory angina, uncontrolled hypertension, recent myocardial infarction, severe congestive heart failure).

More controversial is a recommendation that testosterone be assessed in men with ED, particularly those who have failed management with PDE5I. This conflicts with the recommendations of some other medical societies; providers will have to discuss this type of testing with individual patients to determine advisability.

A. W. Shindel, MD

Depressive Symptoms and Suicidal Thoughts Among Former Users of Finasteride With Persistent Sexual Side Effects
Irwig MS (George Washington Univ, DC)
J Clin Psychiatry 73:1220-1223, 2012

Objective.—Finasteride, a commonly prescribed medication for male pattern hair loss, has recently been associated with persistent sexual side effects. In addition, depression has recently been added to the product labeling of Propecia (finasteride 1 mg). Finasteride reduces the levels of several neuroactive steroids linked to sexual function and depression. This study assesses depressive symptoms and suicidal thoughts in former users of finasteride who developed persistent sexual side effects despite the discontinuation of finasteride.

Method.—In 2010–2011, former users of finasteride (n = 61) with persistent sexual side effects for ≥ 3 months were administered standardized interviews that gathered demographic information, medical and psychiatric histories, and information on medication use, sexual function, and alcohol consumption. All former users were otherwise healthy men with no baseline sexual dysfunction, chronic medical conditions, current or past psychiatric conditions, or use of oral prescription medications before or during finasteride use. A control group of men (n = 29), recruited from the community, had male pattern hair loss but had never used finasteride and denied any history of psychiatric conditions or use of psychiatric medications. The primary outcomes were the prevalence of depressive symptoms and the prevalence of suicidal thoughts as determined by the Beck Depression Inventory II (BDI-II); all subjects self-administered this questionnaire at the time of the interview or up to 10 months later.

Results.—Rates of depressive symptoms (BDI-II score ≥ 14) were significantly higher in the former finasteride users (75%; 46/61) as compared to the controls (10%; 3/29) ($P < .0001$). Moderate or severe depressive symptoms (BDI-II score ≥ 20) were present in 64% (39/61) of the finasteride group and 0% of the controls. Suicidal thoughts were present in 44% (27/61) of the former finasteride users and in 3% (1/29) of the controls ($P < .0001$).

Conclusions.—Clinicians and potential users of finasteride should be aware of the potential risk of depressive symptoms and suicidal thoughts. The preliminary findings of this study warrant further research with controlled studies.

▶ This interesting study interviews men who used the 5-alpha reductase inhibitor drug finasteride for alopecia with a control group of similarly balding men who had never used the drug.

The limitations of case control for assignment of causality in a study such as this should be readily apparent. One may deduce that men who use a medication to reduce hair loss may have more baseline anxiety/insecurity about appearance; this insecurity may spill over into other domains of life, including sexual function and depression, and lead to significant psychopathology. Self-selection of men who had used finasteride and experienced sexual side effects is another limitation; these men were mostly recruited from a Web site catering to men who attribute their various concerns to Propecia use. Although it would have been more difficult to recruit a study population, it would have been informative to assess depressive symptoms in men who had used finasteride but had not developed sexual dysfunction.

The chicken-and-egg question of finasteride and sexual dysfunction in young men is not solved by this research. However, there is a growing body of evidence that finasteride, through unclear mechanisms, may have negative effects on mental health and sexual function in young men using it for alopecia. Urologists should be aware of publications such as this as well as the large movement of young men with sexual concerns who attribute the onset of their problems to the use of this medication. Further research is required to better understand the true effects of finasteride use in young men.

A. W. Shindel, MD

Sexual dysfunction in people with prodromal or first-episode psychosis
Marques TR, Smith S, Bonaccorso S, et al (King's College London, UK)
Br J Psychiatry 201:131-136, 2012

Background.—Sexual dysfunction is common in psychotic disorder but it is not clear whether it is intrinsic to the development of the illness or secondary to other factors.

Aims.—To compare sexual function in people at ultra-high risk (UHR) of a psychotic disorder, patients with first-episode psychosis predominantly taking antipsychotic drugs and healthy volunteers.

Method.—Sexual function was assessed in a UHR group ($n = 31$), a group with first-episode psychosis ($n = 37$) and a matched control group of healthy volunteers ($n = 56$) using the Sexual Function Questionnaire.

Results.—There was a significant effect of group on sexual function ($P < 0.001$). Sexual dysfunction was evident in 50% of the UHR group, 65% of first-episode patients and 21% of controls. Within the UHR group, sexual dysfunction was more marked in those who subsequently developed psychosis than in those who did not. Across all groups the severity of sexual dysfunction was correlated with the severity of psychotic symptoms ($P < 0.001$). Within the first-episode group there was no significant difference in sexual dysfunction between patients taking prolactin-raising $v.$ prolactin-sparing antipsychotics.

life years. But I will gladly agree with their contention that assessment of sexual health should be included in routine consultations and clinical protocols.

A. W. Shindel, MD

Temporal patterns of selected late toxicities in patients treated with brachytherapy or brachytherapy plus external beam radiation for prostate adenocarcinoma
Buckstein M, Kerns S, Forysthe K, et al (Mount Sinai School of Medicine, NY)
BJU Int 111:E43-E47, 2013

What's known on the subject? and What does the study add?
While the frequencies and severity of late toxicities following prostate bra-chytherapy are well known, less has been published with regard to time to first onset. Several series with limited median follow-up have published time to onset. An extensive analysis of timing to late toxicity following bra-chytherapy for cervical cancer has also been published.

This study is the largest of its kind with the longest median follow-up to capture very late events. It can provide a basis for physician and patient education about when late toxicities can reasonably be expected to occur. The study also shows that a significant amount of erectile dysfunction might be more age related than radiation induced.

Objectives.—• To assess the timing of first onset of late rectal bleeding, late haematuria and erectile dysfunction (ED) following brachytherapy with or without external beam radiation therapy (EBRT) for prostate adenocarcinoma.

• To identify treatment factors and patient characteristics that affect the time to first onset.

Patients and Methods.—• In all, 2046 patients were definitively treated for prostate adenocarcinoma with a full ^{125}I or ^{103}Pd implant or a partial ^{103}Pd implant followed by EBRT with 6 years median follow-up (range 2-17 years).

• Patients were selected for an event of Radiation Therapy Oncology Group (RTOG) grade 2 or greater rectal bleeding, ≥RTOG grade 2 hae-maturia, or a drop in the Mount Sinai Erectile Dysfunction Score from potent to impotent (excluding patients who received androgen deprivation therapy).

• Life tables were generated to calculate actuarial incidence rates of toxicity.

• Wilcoxon rank sum and Cox regression were utilized to identify treat-ment factors affecting time to onset.

Results.—• The incidence rate per 1000 patients for 0—2 years, 2—5 years and 5—10 years following radiation for rectal bleeding is 14.3, 15.9 and 6.5, respectively; for haematuria, 14.0, 8.2 and 1.3, respec-tively; and for ED, 82.4, 48.2 and 42.2, respectively.

• Just 5% of rectal bleeding occurs after 5 years from radiation vs 18% of haematuria cases and 22% of ED.

• On multivariate analysis, time to first onset of rectal bleeding was affected by the addition of EBRT only whereas the time to onset of haematuria was affected by the biological effective dose of the radiation and the addition of EBRT.

• The only factor on multivariate analysis to affect time to onset of ED was the age of the patient at treatment, independent of radiation dose or technique.

Conclusions.—• Unique temporality to first onset of selected toxicities was observed in patients after radioactive implant for prostate adenocarcinoma with or without EBRT.

• Clinicians and patients should be counselled when to expect late toxicities.

• The only factor to affect time to onset of ED is the age of the patient, suggesting possible over-reporting of radiation-induced ED in the light of normal age-related events.

▶ Right or wrong, brachytherapy is perceived by many men to be a less risk-prone therapy for prostate carcinoma. This perception is driven in part by the relative simplicity of the procedure compared with pelvic surgery or an extended course of treatment with external-beam radiation. There are data supportive of brachytherapy as a treatment modality; it must of course be borne in mind that brachytherapy patients tend to be low risk, and, given the current controversy about overtreatment, it may be speculated that some men treated with brachytherapy did not need therapy anyway, so *any* degree of side effect or toxicity is too much.

In this article the authors assessed erectile dysfunction (ED) after brachytherapy in a population of men (with normal erections at baseline) using an institution-specific metric similar to the Erection Hardness Scale. Interestingly (but not unique to this study), men were considered potent even if there was a decline in their erection hardness from "optimal" to "able to have intercourse but suboptimal" or if they became dependent on phosphodiesterase type-5 inhibitors. Certainly this may meet a physician's definition of no ED and might indeed be satisfactory for many patients. But in this era of patient-centered outcomes, it cannot really be argued that a decline from "good" to "adequate" erections is not really preservation of erectile function.

The authors did determine that age was the only predictive factor for onset of ED (mean, 66.9 years vs 69.4 years). It does not appear that there was any adjustment for comorbid vascular diseases known to be associated with ED. The authors go on to conclude that the decline in erectile function after brachytherapy is attributable to aging rather than treatment, this despite the fact that the highest incident rate of ED was in the first 2 years after treatment.

It does not necessarily follow that these men were destined for ED irrespective of brachytherapy treatment. It cannot be argued that any treatment modality for prostate cancer offers the chance for physiologic improvement in sexual function, so the importance of discussing ED risk with patients before prostate cancer treatment remains. This study does not negate the existing data that brachytherapy is indeed a risk factor for ED.

A. W. Shindel, MD

Irbesartan promotes erection recovery after nerve-sparing radical retropubic prostatectomy: a retrospective long-term analysis
Segal RL, Bivalacqua TJ, Burnett AL (Johns Hopkins Med Institutions, Baltimore, MD)
BJU Int 110:1782-1786, 2012

Objective.—• To evaluate retrospectively the potential benefit of administering irbesartan, an angiotensin-receptor blocker, to improve erectile function (EF) recovery after nerve-sparing radical retropubic prostatectomy (RRP).

Patients and Methods.—• Before surgery potent patients who underwent nerve-sparing RRP between April and December 2009 elected to start daily oral irbesartan 300 mg on postoperative day 1 ($n = 17$). A contemporaneously clinically matched cohort consisting of patients who declined irbesartan use served as the control group ($n = 12$).

• Postoperative 'on demand' use of erectile aids (phosphodiesterase type 5 [PDE5] inhibitors and intracavernous injections) was adopted.

• Potency was monitored by the administration of International Index of Erectile Function-5 (IIEF-5) questionnaires before surgery and at early (3 months) and long-term (12 and 24 months) postoperative intervals.

• Stretched penile length (SPL) was measured both immediately and 3 months after surgery.

Results.—• EF status was no different between groups at baseline ($P > 0.05$).

• While the IIEF-5 scores at 24 months after surgery were statistically similar between the two groups (control = 15.2 ± 2.0, irbesartan = 14.1 ± 3.1, $P = 0.77$), at 12 months the IIEF-5 scores of the irbesartan group were significantly higher than those of the control group (14 ± 2.6 vs. 7.2 ± 1.6, $P < 0.05$).

• The proportional loss of SPL after RRP was less in the irbesartan than in the control group at 3 months ($-0.9 \pm 1.5\%$ vs -5.6 ± 1.5, $P < 0.05$).

Conclusion.—• Regular irbesartan use after nerve-sparing RRP in patients with normal preoperative erectile function could improve EF recovery after surgery and mitigate early loss of SPL.

*Study Type.—*Therapy (retrospective cohort).

*Level of Evidence.—*2b.

*What's Known on the Subject? and What Does the Study Add?.—*Erectile dysfunction following radical prostatectomy (RP) is among the most common and dreaded adverse effects of the surgery. Multiple studies confirm the potential benefit of various drug classes to accelerate the return of erectile function (EF) after RP. There is pre-clinical evidence supporting the use of angiotensin-receptor blockers (ARBs) for this purpose, although this has not been studied in humans.

The present study shows that there may be a benefit in the recovery of EF post-RRP in patients taking a daily dose of irbesartan, an ARB, following RRP. In addition, the use of irbesartan may curb the loss of stretched penile length which occurs postoperatively. Further study in the form of prospective, randomized, placebo-controlled clinical trials are necessary to confirm these findings.

▶ In this retrospective study, a highly respected team of erectile dysfunction (ED) experts evaluate the use of the angiotensin receptor blocker (ARB) drug irbesartan taken as a penile rehabilitation agent compared with men who declined this treatment. There is evidence that ARBs have neutral or even beneficial effects on erectile function, particularly relative to other antihypertensives such as thiazides or beta-blockers. Although there was no difference at the final time point of 2 years, men taking the drug had better International Index of Erectile Function-erectile function scores at the 12-month time point. Penile stretch length was reportedly preserved in the treatment group, but interestingly these data are reported only for the 3-month time point, not for later time intervals.

Like many studies of postprostatectomy penile rehabilitation, this research is hampered by lack of randomization at initiation of the trial. There were some disparities in comorbid conditions at baseline; specifically, hypertension and tobacco use were more common in the treated men and diabetes more common in the control men, although the absolute number differences were small. Hence, one must consider patient motivation and health as very relevant confounding factors when interpreting these results. The difference in hypertension may be particularly salient given the antihypertensive nature of ARB.

These data are interesting and this topic merits further investigation in a randomized, controlled trial.

A. W. Shindel, MD

13 Hypogonadism

Testosterone Therapy in Men With Prostate Cancer: Scientific and Ethical Considerations
Morgentaler A (Harvard Med School, Boston, MA)
J Urol 189:S26-S33, 2013

Purpose.—Pertinent literature regarding the potential use of testosterone therapy in men with prostate cancer is reviewed and synthesized.

Materials and Methods.—A literature search was performed of English language publications on testosterone administration in men with a known history of prostate cancer and investigation of the effects of androgen concentrations on prostate parameters, especially prostate specific antigen.

Results.—The prohibition against the use of testosterone therapy in men with a history of prostate cancer is based on a model that assumes the androgen sensitivity of prostate cancer extends throughout the range of testosterone concentrations. Although it is clear that prostate cancer is exquisitely sensitive to changes in serum testosterone at low concentrations, there is considerable evidence that prostate cancer growth becomes androgen indifferent at higher concentrations. The most likely mechanism for this loss of androgen sensitivity at higher testosterone concentrations is the finite capacity of the androgen receptor to bind androgen. This saturation model explains why serum testosterone appears unrelated to prostate cancer risk in the general population and why testosterone administration in men with metastatic prostate cancer causes rapid progression in castrated but not hormonally intact men. Worrisome features of prostate cancer such as high Gleason score, extracapsular disease and biochemical recurrence after surgery have been reported in association with low but not high testosterone. In 6 uncontrolled studies results of testosterone therapy have been reported after radical prostatectomy, external beam radiation therapy or brachytherapy. In a total of 111 men 2 (1.8%) biochemical recurrences were observed. Anecdotal evidence suggests that testosterone therapy does not necessarily cause increased prostate specific antigen even in men with untreated prostate cancer.

Conclusions.—Although no controlled studies have been performed to date to document the safety of testosterone therapy in men with prostate cancer, the limited available evidence suggests that such treatment may not pose an undue risk of prostate cancer recurrence or progression.

▶ Testosterone replacement in men who are at risk for prostate cancer, who have untreated prostate cancer, or who have apparently successfully treated prostate cancer, is controversial. There is clearly an upside in terms of quality of life in men with symptomatic hypogonadism, but this must be balanced against the risks associated with exacerbating known or unknown prostate cancer. This article addresses the controversy and reviews much of the relevant data currently available. On balance, it seems that testosterone replacement will be safe if close follow-up is maintained.

G. L. Andriole, Jr, MD

14 STD

Quadrivalent Human Papillomavirus Vaccine Effectiveness: A Swedish National Cohort Study

Leval A, Herweijer E, Ploner A, et al (Karolinska Institutet, Stockholm, Sweden; et al)

J Natl Cancer Inst 105:469-474, 2013

Background.—Incidence of condyloma, or genital warts (GW), is the earliest possible disease outcome to measure when assessing the effectiveness of human papillomavirus (HPV) vaccination strategies. Efficacy trials that follow prespecified inclusion and exclusion criteria may not be fully generalizable to real-life HPV vaccination programs, which target a broader segment of the population. We assessed GW incidence after on-demand vaccination with quadrivalent HPV vaccine using individual-level data from the entire Swedish population.

Methods.—An open cohort of girls and women aged 10 to 44 years living in Sweden between 2006 and 2010 (N >2.2 million) was linked to multiple population registers to identify incident GW in relation to HPV vaccination. For vaccine effectiveness, incidence rate ratios of GW were estimated using time-to-event analyses with adjustment for attained age and parental education level, stratifying on age at first vaccination.

Results. A total of 124 000 girls and women were vaccinated between 2006 and 2010. Girls and women with at least one university-educated parent were 15 times more likely to be vaccinated before age 20 years than girls and women whose parents did not complete high school (relative risk ratio = 15.45, 95% confidence interval [CI] = 14.65 to 16.30). Among those aged older than 20 years, GW rates declined among the unvaccinated, suggesting that HPV vaccines were preferentially used by women at high risk of GW. Vaccination effectiveness was 76% (95% CI = 73% to 79%) among those who received three doses of the vaccine with their first dose before age 20 years. Vaccine effectiveness was highest in girls vaccinated before age 14 years (effectiveness = 93%, 95% CI = 73% to 98%).

Conclusions.—Young age at first vaccination is imperative for maximizing quadrivalent HPV vaccine effectiveness.

▶ Quadrivalent human papillomavirus (HPV) vaccine (types 6, 11, 16, and 18) was first approved for use in females in 2006. It protects nearly 100% of naïve females and decreases the incidence of all genital warts to 80%. The clinical trials may not reflect real-life efficacy because the study population is typically highly selected.

This population-based study shows that efficacy is related to age at vaccination (a surrogate for exposure to HPV). Long-term follow-up should show a decreased incidence of HPV-related cervical dysplasia and cancer. There is little efficacy in patients over age 22. Presumably, those with high-risk behavior were vaccinated, but the vaccine does not eliminate the virus in those already exposed.

Although the study shows excellent efficacy from a preventive health perspective, the utility is not optimal because a large population of females (those with lower socioeconomic status) were not vaccinated.

D. E. Coplen, MD

15 Renal Tumors

Diagnosis and Prognosis

Utility of the RENAL nephrometry scoring system in the real world: predicting surgeon operative preference and complication risk
Rosevear HM, Gellhaus PT, Lightfoot AJ, et al (Univ of Iowa)
BJU Int 100:700 706, 2012

Objective.—• To evaluate the utility of the RENAL scoring system in predicting operative approach and risk of complications. The RENAL nephrometry scoring system is designed to allow comparison of renal masses based on the radiological features of (R)adius, (E)xophytic/endophytic, (N)earness to collecting system, (A)nterior/posterior and (L)ocation relative to polar lines.

Methods.—• A retrospective review of all patients at a single institution undergoing radical nephrectomy (RN) or partial nephrectomy (PN) for a renal mass between July 2007 and May 2010 was carried out.

• Preoperative RENAL score was calculated for each patient. Surgical approach and operative outcomes were then compared with the RENAL score.

Results.—• In all, 249 patients underwent either RN (158) or PN (91) with average RENAL scores of 8.9 and 6.3, respectively ($P < 0.001$).

• Patients who underwent RN were more likely to have hilar tumours (64% vs 10%, $P < 0.001$) than patients who underwent PN, but were no more likely to have posteriorly located tumours (50% each).

• There were more complications among patients with RN (58%) vs patients with PN (42%, $P = 0.02$).

• RENAL scores were higher in patients with PN who developed complications than in patients with PN who did not develop complications (6.9 vs 6.0, $P = 0.02$), with no difference noted among patients with RN developing complications (8.9 vs 8.9, $P = 0.99$).

Conclusion.—• The RENAL system accurately predicted surgeon operative preference and risk of complications for patients undergoing PN.

▶ Kutikov and Uzzo[1] created the nephrometry score to standardize the classification of renal masses based on anatomical complexity. The acronym RENAL details the 5 components of complexity—*R*adius, *E*xophytic versus endophytic properties, *N*earness to the collecting system or renal sinus, *A* is noted as anterior, posterior, or other, and Location to the polar line—and each is given a numeric value ranging from 1 through 3 corresponding to increasing complexity. Hilar masses touching the main renal artery or vein are given a special hilar designation. The sum of the 4 numeric properties characterizes the lesion as low (4 to 6), moderate (7 to 9), or high complexity (10 to 12). An increasing renal score has previously been associated with urine leak,[2] higher estimated blood loss, longer warm ischemia times, and a longer length of hospital stay in patients undergoing partial nephrectomies.[3]

The authors performed a retrospective assignment of nephrometry scores for 249 patients who underwent a radical nephrectomy (RN) or partial nephrectomy (PN) between July 2007 and May 2010. The preoperative characteristics of the 2 groups were similar with the exception of the PN patients having a propensity toward a younger age (54 vs 60 years). The RENAL score was found to have predictive value regarding choice of surgical approach. Of the 5 RENAL categories, only the endophytic versus exophytic properties and anterior versus posterior location had no bearing on the decision to perform PN versus RN in the laparoscopic groups. A trend toward open RN compared to open PN was seen with higher RENAL category scores with the exception of the anterior versus posterior location.

The rate of complication was greater in the RN group compared to the PN group (58% vs 42%). Patients undergoing laparoscopic PN had higher RENAL scores in the complication groups compared to the noncomplication group. Patients who underwent RN without complications had similar nephrometry scores to patients who underwent RN with complications.

This study was limited by its retrospective approach that could underreport complications. At the time of publication, the mean follow-up time was only 6.1 and 8.3 months for PN and RN, respectively. Unfortunately, at such short intervals, survival data were not yet available. Future data will likely find more correlations with nephrometry scores and other perioperative and postoperative data.

J. M. Mobley, MD

References

1. Kutikov A, Uzzo RG. The R.E.N.A.L nephrometry score: a comprehensive standardized system for quantitating renal tumor size, location and depth. *J Urol.* 2009;182:844-853.
2. Bruner B, Breau RH, Lohse CM, Leibovich BC, Blute ML. Renal nephrometry score is associated with urine leak after partial nephrectomy. *BJU Int.* 2011; 108:67-72.
3. Hayn MH, Schwaab T, Underwood W, Kim HL. RENAL nephrometry score predicts surgical outcomes of laparoscopic partial nephrectomy. *BJU Int.* 2010; 108:879-881.

RENAL Nephrometry Score Predicts Surgery Type Independent of Individual Surgeon's Use of Nephron-Sparing Surgery

Tobert CM, Kahnoski RJ, Thompson DE, et al (Spectrum Health Hosp System, Grand Rapids, MI; Michigan State Univ, Grand Rapids)

Urology 80:157-161, 2012

Objective.—To evaluate whether surgeon factors, such as training and experience, have a strong impact on selection of surgical approach for treating renal cancers. Nephron-sparing surgery (NSS) has become the reference standard for tumors that are amenable to such an approach. Tumor size and configuration are important predictors of usage of NSS. The RENAL nephrometry score (RNS) has been developed to standardize reporting of tumor complexity, but the performance of this method within individual surgeons' practices, particularly in the community-based setting, has not been evaluated previously.

Methods.—Clinical data and RNS were collected retrospectively for 300 cases performed by 5 different surgeons with varying NSS usage rates (31-74%).

Results.—Mean RNS for patients undergoing NSS (6.0) and radical nephrectomy (RN) (9.3) differed significantly ($P < .0001$), as did tumor size (2.8 vs 6.3 cm, $P < .0001$). RNS was a better predictor of surgery type ($R^2 = .55$) than was tumor size ($R^2 = .43$) for all 5 surgeons. In univariable analysis, individual surgeon, surgery year, glomerular filtration rate, tumor size, RNS, and each RNS component predicted NSS vs RN (each $P < .05$). In multivariable analysis, surgeon, tumor size, exophytic amount, and nearness to collecting system were independent predictors of NSS usage ($P < .001$).

Conclusion.—Despite significant variation in NSS usage by individual surgeons at a community-based health system, RNS appears to be valid for both low and high usage. With increasing usage of NSS worldwide, RNS appears to reflect current patterns and may inform future practice for surgeons of all backgrounds.

▶ This article evaluates the utility of the RENAL (*R*adius, *E*xophytic/endophytic, *N*earness to collecting system, *A*nterior/posterior, and *L*ocation) nephrometry score in predicting usage of nephron-sparing surgery. The study finds that the utilization of nephron-sparing surgery correlated more closely with the nephrometry score than with tumor size alone, and that the mean nephrometry score was higher in patients undergoing radical nephrectomy compared with those undergoing nephron-sparing surgery. Furthermore, the study demonstrates that several individual components of the RENAL nephrometry scoring system, including tumor size, exophytic component, and nearness to the collecting system, were independent predictors of nephron-sparing surgery utilization on multivariate analysis.

Since its inception as a comprehensive standardized system for quantitating renal tumor size, location, and depth,[1] the nephrometry scoring system has been widely utilized as a tool for assessing tumor complexity in a variety of clinical scenarios. Yet few studies have externally validated the utility of this instrument in predicting surgical outcomes. A recent Mayo Clinic study of 95 patients who underwent surgical treatment for solid renal masses validated the interreviewer reproducibility of the nephrometry scoring system among 6 independent reviewers and the ability of higher nephrometry scores to predict increased risk of distant metastasis and death from renal cell carcinoma.[2] A study including 249 patients by Rosevear and colleagues[3] demonstrated that higher RENAL nephrometry scores predicted increased complication rates in patients undergoing partial nephrectomy and an increased propensity for radical nephrectomy relative to partial nephrectomy. This analysis provides further validation of the utility of the nephrometry scoring system in predicting the usage of nephron-sparing surgery, thus supporting its role in clinical decision making.

Y. S. Tanagho, MD, MPH

References

1. Kutikov A, Uzzo RG. The R.E.N.A.L. nephrometry score: a comprehensive standardized system for quantitating renal tumor size, location and depth. *J Urol.* 2009;182:844-853.
2. Weight CJ, Atwell TD, Fazzio RT, et al. A multidisciplinary evaluation of interreviewer agreement of the nephrometry score and the prediction of long-term outcomes. *J Urol.* 2011;186:1223-1228.
3. Rosevear HM, Gellhaus PT, Lightfoot AJ, et al. Utility of the RENAL nephrometry scoring system in the real world: predicting surgeon operative preference and complication risk. *BJU Int.* 2012;109:700-705.

Partial Nephrectomy

Functional Analysis of Elective Nephron-sparing Surgery vs Radical Nephrectomy for Renal Tumors Larger than 4 cm

Roos FC, Brenner W, Thomas C, et al (Johannes Gutenberg Univ, Mainz, Germany)
Urology 79:607-614, 2012

Objective.—To preserve renal function, nephron sparing surgery (NSS) for renal tumors should be performed. Little is known about perioperative morbidity and long-term functional outcome of patients after elective NSS compared with radical nephrectomy (RN) in renal tumors >4 cm.

Materials and Methods.—Eight-hundred twenty-nine patients were treated with either RN (n = 641) or NSS (n = 188) for renal tumors >4 cm. After pairing the cohort for age, grading, TNM, size, gender, and preoperative renal function and excluding patients with imperative indication and metastases, 247 patients remained for functional analysis. Serum creatinine (SCr) values were used to estimate glomerular filtration rate (eGFR) via Modification of Diet in Renal Disease. Chronic kidney disease (CKD) was defined as eGFR <60 mL/min/1.73 m^2 and regression analyses were used to identify clinical risk factors for CKD and perioperative complications stratified by the Clavien-Dindo score.

Results.—The Charlson comorbidity index was similar between patients undergoing NSS (n = 101) and RN (n = 146) (*P* =.583). The complication rates did not differ significantly between both groups (*P* =.091). Age (OR 0.94, *P* =.009), ASA score 3 + 4 (OR 3.55, *P* =.004), RN (OR 10.75, *P* < .001), and preoperative eGFR (OR 1.06, *P* < .001) were independent risk factors for developing CKD postoperatively, whereas tumor size had no impact (OR 1.01, *P* =.245). Overall survival was comparable between the groups (*P* =.896).

Conclusion.—Although overall survival was similar, patients undergoing RN for renal tumors >4 cm had a significantly higher risk of developing CKD than patients treated with NSS. Complication rate did not differ significantly between both groups, even for tumors >7 cm. Our findings support elective NSS for tumors >4 cm, whenever NSS is technically feasible for maintaining renal function.

▶ This article compares the perioperative morbidity of elective partial nephrectomy versus radical nephrectomy for tumors greater than 4 cm and evaluates the relative likelihood of long-term development of chronic kidney disease using these alternative surgical approaches in a multivariate logistic regression model. The study demonstrates no difference in complication rates between the 2 surgical approaches, while providing evidence of an advantage in long-term renal functional preservation favoring the nephron-sparing approach.

Current American Urological Association guidelines endorse partial nephrectomy as the standard of care for the management of T1a renal tumors and as an acceptable treatment alternative to radical nephrectomy in patients with T1b renal tumors.[1] This study adds to a growing body of literature that suggests that nephron-sparing surgery is associated with decreased morbidity relative to radical nephrectomy.[2-5] Although nephron-sparing surgery was not associated with a survival benefit in this study, other observational studies do suggest that nephron-sparing surgery may indeed result in improved overall survival relative to radical nephrectomy.[4,5] Nevertheless, level 1 evidence demonstrating a survival benefit favoring nephron-sparing surgery is notably lacking. Observational studies, including this study, cannot entirely eliminate the potential for confounding and selection bias and, hence, do not preclude the need for future randomized trials comparing morbidity and mortality in patients undergoing nephron sparing surgery versus those undergoing radical nephrectomy.

Y. S. Tanagho, MD, MPH

References

1. American Urological Association Education and Research (AUA) Guidelines. "Guidelines for Management of the Clinical Stage I Renal Mass." Renal Mass Clinical Panel Chairs: Novick AC (Chair), Campbell SC (Co-Chair). www.auanet.org/content/media/renalmass09.pdf. Accessed March 21, 2012.
2. Go AS, Chertow GM, Fan D, McCulloch CE, Hsu CY. Chronic kidney disease and the risks of death, cardiovascular events, and hospitalization. *N Engl J Med.* 2004; 351:1296-1305.
3. Huang WC, Levey AS, Serio AM, et al. Chronic kidney disease after nephrectomy in patients with renal cortical tumors: a retrospective cohort study. *Lancet Oncol.* 2006;7:735-740.

4. Thompson RH, Boorjian SA, Lohse CM, et al. Radical nephrectomy for pT1a renal masses may be associated with decreased overall survival compared with partial nephrectomy. *J Urol.* 2008;179:468-471.
5. Weight CJ, Lieser G, Larson BT, et al. Partial nephrectomy is associated with improved overall survival compared to radical nephrectomy in patients with unanticipated benign renal tumors. *Eur Urol.* 2010;58:293-298.

'Zero ischaemia', sutureless laparoscopic partial nephrectomy for renal tumours with a low nephrometry score

Simone G, Papalia R, Guaglianone S, et al ('Regina Elena' Natl Cancer Inst, Rome, Italy)
BJU Int 110:124-130, 2012

Objective.—• To describe the technique and report the results of 'zero ischaemia', sutureless laparoscopic partial nephrectomy (LPN) for renal tumours with a low nephrometry score.

Patients and Methods.—• Between August 2003 and January 2010, data from 101 consecutive patients who underwent 'zero ischaemia', sutureless LPN were collected in a prospectively maintained database.

• Inclusion criteria were tumour size ≤4 cm, predominant exophytic growth and intraparenchymal depth ≤1.5 cm, with a minimum distance of 5 mm from the urinary collecting system.

• Hilar vessels were not isolated, tumour dissection was performed with 10-mm LigaSure TM (Covidien, Boulder, CO, USA) and haemostasis was performed with coagulation and biological haemostatic agents without reconstructing the renal parenchyma.

• Clinical, perioperative and follow-up data were collected prospectively, and modifications of functional outcome variables were analysed using the paired Wilcoxon test.

Results.—• The median (range) tumour size was 2.4 (1.5−4) cm, and the median (range) intraparenchymal depth was 0.7 (0.4−1.4) cm.

• Hilar clamping was not necessary in any patient, and suture was performed in four patients to ensure complete haemostasis. The median (range) operation duration was 60 (45−160) min, and median (range) intraoperative blood loss was 100 (20−240) mL.

• Postoperative complications included fever ($n = 4$), low urinary output ($n = 3$) and haematoma, which was treated conservatively ($n = 2$). The median (range) hospital stay was 3 (2−5) days. The pathologist reported 30 benign tumours and renal cell carcinoma in 71 cases (pT1a in 69 patients, and pT1b in two patients).

• At a median follow-up of 57 months, one patient underwent radical nephrectomy for ipsilateral recurrence. The 1-year median (range) decrease of split renal function at renal scintigraphy was 1 (0−5) %.

Conclusions.—• Zero ischaemia LPN is a reasonable approach to treating small and peripheral tumours, and a sutureless procedure is feasible in most cases.

- This technique has a low complication rate and provides excellent functional outcome without impairing oncological results.

▶ This article demonstrates the feasibility and safety of performing laparoscopic partial nephrectomy without renal hilar dissection or clamping using a sutureless technique for select tumors of low nephrometry score. In view of mounting evidence highlighting the importance of renal preservation,[1-4] this study also evaluated the renal functional outcomes of this off-clamp technique and demonstrated minimal decrease in the split renal function of the affected kidney at a median 1-year follow-up.

The significant increase in incidentally discovered small renal masses,[5] in the absence of reliable molecular markers predicting the natural history or clinical significance of such lesions, places additional impetus on the surgeon to minimize the morbidity associated with extirpative renal surgery. Insofar as techniques for achieving renal hypothermia during minimally invasive nephron-sparing surgery have failed to gain widespread clinical application, zero ischemia partial nephrectomy represents an attractive surgical alternative, effectively eliminating ischemic injury during minimally invasive nephron-sparing surgery. Nevertheless, additional studies are needed to compare the renal functional outcomes of off-clamp versus clamped partial nephrectomy to demonstrate any putative advantage in renal preservation favoring the off-clamp technique. Future studies may also incorporate evaluation of biomarkers of ischemic renal injury in the comparative assessment of clamped versus off-clamp partial nephrectomy. Although a large, randomized, prospective study comparing the renal functional outcomes of clamped versus off-clamp partial nephrectomy is indicated, given the considerable need for careful patient selection during initial cases of off-clamp partial nephrectomy, such a study is best reserved until more extensive experience with the off-clamp technique has been attained.

Y. S. Tanagho, MD, MPH

References

1. Go AS, Chertow GM, Fan D, McCulloch CE, Hsu CY. Chronic kidney disease and the risks of death, cardiovascular events, and hospitalization. *N Engl J Med.* 2004; 351:1296-1305.
2. Huang WC, Levey AS, Serio AM, et al. Chronic kidney disease after nephrectomy in patients with renal cortical tumors: a retrospective cohort study. *Lancet Oncol.* 2006;7:735-740.
3. Thompson RH, Boorjian SA, Lohse CM, et al. Radical nephrectomy for pT1a renal masses may be associated with decreased overall survival compared with partial nephrectomy. *J Urol.* 2008;179:468-471.
4. Weight CJ, Lieser G, Larson BT, et al. Partial nephrectomy is associated with improved overall survival compared to radical nephrectomy in patients with unanticipated benign renal tumors. *Eur Urol.* 2010;58:293-298.
5. Kane CJ, Mallin K, Ritchey J, Cooperberg MR, Carroll PR. Renal cell cancer stage migration: analysis of the National Cancer Data Base. *Cancer.* 2008;113:78-83.

Trends in the use of of nephron–sparing surgery (NSS) at an Australian tertiary referral centre: an analysis of surgical decision–making using the R.E.N.A.L. nephrometry scoring system

Satasivam P, Rajarubendra N, Chia PH, et al (The Austin Hosp, Heidelberg, Victoria, Australia)
BJU Int 109:1341-1344, 2012

Objective.—• To examine recent trends in the use of nephron-sparing surgery (NSS) at our centre. Specifically, we sought to examine the process of surgical decision-making by applying the R.E.N.A.L. nephrometry scoring system to assess the complexity of lesions for which surgery was undertaken.

Patients and Methods.—• We performed a retrospective review of renal masses treated by surgery from January 2005 to December 2009, including 79 RN and 70 NSS.

• CT images were available for analysis in 50 patients within each group.

• Lesions were scored on the basis of their complexity using the R.E.N.A.L. nephrometry scoring system developed by Kutikov and Uzzo.

Results.—• There was no difference in age between patients undergoing RN and NSS (median age 61 vs 60 years).

• RN was performed for significantly larger lesions (mean [sd] 68 [9] vs 29 [2] mm, $P < 0.05$) of predominantly moderate and high complexity (12% low, 56% moderate, 32% high).

• NSS was primarily used for low-complexity lesions, but included four (8%) moderate-complexity lesions in the final 2 years of the study.

• The use of NSS increased from 28.6% of cases in 2005 to 60.0% of cases in 2009, which mirrored the increase in the proportion of operations performed for low-complexity lesions (22.2% low-complexity in 2005 to 70.6% in 2009, $P < 0.01$ for trend).

Conclusions.—• The increasing use of NSS at our institution mirrored the increasing treatment of low-complexity renal lesions.

• This may reflect an increased detection and referral of such lesions, or a shift towards treatment of lesions that in the past would have been under surveillance.

• Practice at our centre reflects a shifting paradigm towards preferential use of NSS for the treatment of suitable renal masses.

▶ This article examines trends in the utilization of nephron-sparing surgery at an Australian tertiary referral center. The article demonstrates that decreased tumor size and lower tumor complexity correlate with increased utilization of nephron-sparing surgery and, furthermore, that the use of nephron-sparing surgery increased over the time course of this study. The authors attribute the shifting paradigm toward preferential use of nephron-sparing surgery to the increasing detection of lower-complexity tumors on abdominal imaging as well as an increasing propensity for surgical management of small tumors, which in the past may have undergone surveillance.

Although the authors' assertion that increased incidental detection of small renal masses contributes to the increased utilization of nephron-sparing surgery is plausible, mounting evidence highlighting the importance of nephron-sparing surgery in reducing the incidence of chronic kidney disease as well as cardiovascular morbidity and mortality[1-4] has certainly contributed to the increased utilization of nephron-sparing surgery independent of the stage migration favoring smaller, less complex tumors highlighted in this study. This study would have benefited from an evaluation of contemporary trends in the utilization of partial nephrectomy that controls for tumor size, complexity, and stage at presentation. An evaluation of discrepancies in the utilization of nephron-sparing surgery at high-volume, tertiary centers of excellence versus general community practices is also of interest in light of the significant underutilization of nephron-sparing surgery that has been demonstrated in numerous studies.[5,6]

Y. S. Tanagho, MD, MPH

References

1. Thompson R, Boorjiana S, Lohseb C, et al. Radical nephrectomy for pT1a renal masses may be associated with decreased overall survival compared with partial nephrectomy. *J Urol.* 2008;179:468-473.
2. Becker F, Siemer S, Humke U, Hack M, Ziegler M, Stöckle M. Elective nephron sparing surgery should become standard treatment for small unilateral renal cell carcinoma: long-term survival data of 216 patients. *Eur Urol.* 2006;49:308-313.
3. Huang WC, Elkin EB, Levey AS, Jang TL, Russo P. Partial nephrectomy versus radical nephrectomy in patients with small renal tumors—is there a difference in mortality and cardiovascular outcomes? *J Urol.* 2009;181:55-61.
4. Weight CJ, Lieser G, Larson BT, et al. Partial nephrectomy is associated with improved overall survival compared to radical nephrectomy in patients with unanticipated benign renal tumours. *Eur Urol.* 2010;58:293-298.
5. Patel SG, Penson DF, Pabla B, et al. National trends in the use of partial nephrectomy: a rising tide that has not lifted all boats. *J Urol.* 2012;187:816-821.
6. Kim SP, Shah ND, Weight CJ, et al. Contemporary trends in nephrectomy for renal cell carcinoma in the United States: results from a population based cohort. *J Urol.* 2011;186:1779-1785.

16 Prostate Cancer

Screening

Quality-of-Life Effects of Prostate-Specific Antigen Screening

Heijnsdijk FAM, Wever EM, Auvinen A, et al (Erasmus Med Ctr, Rotterdam, the Netherlands; Tampere School of Health Sciences, Finland; et al)
N Engl J Med 367:595-605, 2012

Background.—After 11 years of follow-up, the European Randomized Study of Screening for Prostate Cancer (ERSPC) reported a 29% reduction in prostate-cancer mortality among men who underwent screening for prostate-specific antigen (PSA) levels. However, the extent to which harms to quality of life resulting from overdiagnosis and treatment counterbalance this benefit is uncertain.

Methods.—On the basis of ERSPC follow-up data, we used Microsimulation Screening Analysis (MISCAN) to predict the number of prostate cancers, treatments, deaths, and quality-adjusted life-years (QALYs) gained after the introduction of PSA screening. Various screening strategies, efficacies, and quality-of-life assumptions were modeled.

Results.—Per 1000 men of all ages who were followed for their entire life span, we predicted that annual screening of men between the ages of 55 and 69 years would result in nine fewer deaths from prostate cancer (28% reduction), 14 fewer men receiving palliative therapy (35% reduction), and a total of 73 life-years gained (average, 8.4 years per prostate-cancer death avoided). The number of QALYs that were gained was 56 (range, −21 to 97), a reduction of 23% from unadjusted life-years gained. To prevent one prostate-cancer death, 98 men would need to be screened and 5 cancers would need to be detected. Screening of all men between the ages of 55 and 74 would result in more life-years gained (82) but the same number of QALYs (56).

Conclusions.—The benefit of PSA screening was diminished by loss of QALYs owing to postdiagnosis long-term effects. Longer follow-up data from both the ERSPC and quality-of-life analyses are essential before universal recommendations regarding screening can be made. (Funded by the Netherlands Organization for Health Research and Development and others.)

▶ The problem with models is that they are only as good as the assumptions and data that are put into them. The strength of this study is that the data placed into the model are from the largest randomized trial of prostate-specific antigen screening. The model demonstrates that to prevent 1 prostate cancer death, 98 men would need to be screened and 5 cancers would need to be detected. Importantly, quality of life would be improved for the population as a whole. If one screened a younger population (55 to 69 years of age), not only is there an improvement in life expectancy, but quality of life is also improved. Now there is clearly a cost. The model assumes that there is almost a 50% overdiagnosis rate of prostate cancer. This means that many individual patients will be treated unnecessarily. Once again, the risk of screening and treatment needs to be balanced against the risk of adverse events. I suspect that introduction of active surveillance will improve the quality of life for all men with newly diagnosed prostate cancer. Most of the loss of quality of life is not from the biopsy, but rather from the treatment. Embracing active surveillance would therefore likely improve quality of life findings in this model and more strongly favor screening.

A. S. Kibel, MD

Serum Isoform [−2]proPSA Derivatives Significantly Improve Prediction of Prostate Cancer at Initial Biopsy in a Total PSA Range of 2−10 ng/ml: A Multicentric European Study
Lazzeri M, Haese A, de la Taille A, et al (San Raffaele Scientific Inst, Milan, Italy; Univ Clinic Hamburg-Eppendorf, Germany; APHP Mondor Hosp, Créteil, France; et al)
Eur Urol 63:986-994, 2013

Background.—Strategies to reduce prostate-specific antigen (PSA)—driven prostate cancer (PCa) overdiagnosis and overtreatment seem to be necessary.

Objective.—To test the accuracy of serum isoform [−2]proPSA (p2PSA) and its derivatives, percentage of p2PSA to free PSA (fPSA; %p2PSA) and the Prostate Health Index (PHI)—called *index tests*—in discriminating between patients with and without PCa.

Design, Setting, and Participants.—This was an observational, prospective cohort study of patients from five European urologic centers with a total PSA (tPSA) range of 2−10 ng/ml who were subjected to initial prostate biopsy for suspected PCa.

Outcome Measurements and Statistical Analysis.—The primary end point was to evaluate the specificity, sensitivity, and diagnostic accuracy of index tests in determining the presence of PCa at prostate biopsy in comparison to tPSA, fPSA, and percentage of fPSA to tPSA (%fPSA) (standard tests) and the number of prostate biopsies that could be spared using these tests. Multivariable logistic regression models were complemented by predictive accuracy analysis and decision curve analysis.

Results and Limitations.—Of >646 patients, PCa was diagnosed in 264 (40.1%). Median tPSA (5.7 vs 5.8 ng/ml; $p = 0.942$) and p2PSA (15.0 vs 14.7 pg/ml) did not differ between groups; conversely, median fPSA (0.7 vs 1 ng/ml; $p < 0.001$), %fPSA (0.14 vs 0.17; $p < 0.001$), %p2PSA (2.1 vs 1.6; $p < 0.001$), and PHI (48.2 vs 38; $p < 0.001$) did differ significantly between men with and without PCa. In multivariable logistic regression models, p2PSA, %p2PSA, and PHI significantly increased the accuracy of the base multivariable model by 6.4%, 5.6%, and 6.4%, respectively (all $p < 0.001$). At a PHI cut-off of 27.6, a total of 100 (15.5%) biopsies could have been avoided. The main limitation is that cases were selected on the basis of their initial tPSA values.

Conclusions.—In patients with a tPSA range of 2–10 ng/ml, %p2PSA and PHI are the strongest predictors of PCa at initial biopsy and are significantly more accurate than tPSA and %fPSA

Trial Registration.—The study is registered at http://www.controlled-trials.com, ref. ISRCTN04707454.

▶ There is an urgent need to improve prostate-specific antigen (PSA)–based screening by reducing negative biopsies, and use of [−2]proPSA and the prostate health index seems to be a step in the right direction. Use of these tools can reduce many negative biopsies or biopsies that detect only Gleason 6 cancer while missing very few aggressive cancers. Other Kallikrein markers also may be beneficial in this regard. Avoiding negative biopsies is a real plus given the increasing risk of biopsy-related infections and perhaps mortality.

G. L. Andriole, Jr, MD

Critical role of prostate biopsy mortality In the number of years of life gained and lost within a prostate cancer screening programme
Boniol M, Boyle P, Autier P, et al (International Prevention Res Inst (IPRI), Lyon, France; et al)
BJU Int 110:1648-1653, 2012

What's known on the subject? and What does the study add?
The efficacy of prostate cancer screening using PSA testing is still being debated, with conflicting results in randomized trials.
The study shows that, even using the hypothesis most favourable to prostate cancer screening with PSA, the net number of years of life does not favour screening.

Objective.—● To evaluate the impact of the implementation a prostate-specific antigen (PSA) screening programme using the European Randomized Study of Screening for Prostate Cancer (ERSPC) results and taking into account the impact of prostate biopsy and over-treatment on mortality.

TABLE 1.—Calculation of Years of Life Gained and Lost From Prostate Cancer Screening

	Screening	Prostate Cancer	Prostate Cancer Deaths avoided
Frequency from ERSPC 2012 (a)	1055	37	1
Years of life gained per death (b)			9.3
Years of life lost per death (c)	17.1	17.1	
Biopsy rate (d)	27%		
Number of biopsies (e) = (a)×(d)	284		
Mortality associated with medical procedure (f)	2 per 1000*	5 per 1000[†]	
Gained in years (g)			9.3 (a) × (b)
Lost in years (h)	9.7 (c) × (e) × (f)	3.2 (a) × (c) × (f)	
Total (g-h) −3.6			

Editor's Note: Please refer to original journal article for full references.
*Gallina et al. [18].
[†]Walz et al. [16].

Materials and Methods.—• We used a model based on the number of years of life gained and lost owing to screening, using data reported in the ERSPC.

• We conducted a critical evaluation of the ERSPC results and of the Swedish arm of the study.

Results.—• Accounting for biopsy-specific mortality and for over-treatment, the balance of number of years of life was negative in the ERSPC study, with an estimated loss of 3.6 years of life per avoided death.

• The number of years of life becomes positive (real gain) only when fewer than 666 screened individuals are required to avoid one death.

• We found that in the Swedish arm of the ERSPC there was a biopsy rate of 40% compared with 27% in the ERSPC overall. The over-treatment rate was also greater with 4.1% compared with 3.4% overall.

• For the last 20 years, there has been a marked difference in prostate cancer-specific mortality between Sweden and the rest of Europe: in 2005, for the age group 65−74 the rate was 140 per 100 000 person years in Sweden and ∼80 per 100 000 for the rest of Europe.

Conclusion.—• Overall, PSA testing in Europe is associated with a loss in years of life and should thus not be recommended.

Study Type.—Therapy (data synthesis).

Level of Evidence.—2b (Table 1).

▶ Table 1 is quite sobering. It suggests the overall mortality benefit of screening for prostate cancer is sensitive to the mortality associated with prostate biopsy, which is sadly increasing. This analysis underscores what a close call prostate-specific antigen−based screening is on a population level.

G. L. Andriole, Jr, MD

Diagnostics

Increasing Hospital Admission Rates for Urological Complications After Transrectal Ultrasound Guided Prostate Biopsy

Nam RK, Saskin R, Lee Y, et al (Sunnybrook Res Inst, Toronto, Ontario, Canada; Inst of Clinical Evaluative Sciences, Toronto, Ontario, Canada; St Michael's Hosp, Toronto, Ontario, Canada; et al)
J Urol 189:S12-S18, 2013

Purpose.—Transrectal ultrasound guided prostate biopsy is widely used to confirm the diagnosis of prostate cancer. The technique has been associated with significant morbidity in a small proportion of patients.

Materials and Methods.—We conducted a population based study of 75,190 men who underwent a transrectal ultrasound guided biopsy in Ontario, Canada, between 1996 and 2005. We used hospital and cancer registry administrative databases to estimate the rates of hospital admission and mortality due to urological complications associated with the procedure.

Results.—Of the 75,190 men who underwent transrectal ultrasound biopsy 33,508 (44.6%) were diagnosed with prostate cancer and 41,682 (55.4%) did not have prostate cancer. The hospital admission rate for urological complications within 30 days of the procedure for men without cancer was 1.9% (781/41,482). The 30-day hospital admission rate increased from 1.0% in 1996 to 4.1% in 2005 (*p* for trend < 0.0001). The majority of hospital admissions (72%) were for infection related reasons. The probability of being admitted to hospital within 30 days of having the procedure increased 4-fold between 1996 and 2005 (OR 3.7, 95% CI 2.0−7.0, *p* < 0.0001). The overall 30-day mortality rate was 0.09% but did not change during the study period.

Conclusions.—The hospital admission rates for complications following transrectal ultrasound guided prostate biopsy have increased dramatically during the last 10 years primarily due to an increasing rate of infection related complications.

▶ Every urologist should be aware of the emerging problem of infection-related complications and, in some studies, of mortality from transrectal ultrasound-guided prostate biopsies. This finding may have a large impact on active surveillance strategies, which, for the most part, rely on serial biopsy to assess whether the initial biopsy underestimated the tumor size or grade or whether the tumor is progressing. Is it time to use more transperineal biopsies or rely on magnetic resonance imaging targeting? Or is modification of the antibiotic prophylaxis regimen all that is needed? Some have also proposed rectal cultures before biopsy to assess for resistant organisms. No doubt better strategies will emerge, but, for now, urologists should scrupulously evaluate men who are to undergo biopsy for any pre-existing urinary tract infection and be certain there is a strong indication for the biopsy.

G. L. Andriole, Jr, MD

Multiparametric Magnetic Resonance Imaging and Ultrasound Fusion Biopsy Detect Prostate Cancer in Patients with Prior Negative Transrectal Ultrasound Biopsies

Vourganti S, Rastinehad A, Yerram NK, et al (Natl Cancer Inst, Bethesda, MD; et al)

J Urol 188:2152-2157, 2012

Purpose.—Patients with negative transrectal ultrasound biopsies and a persistent clinical suspicion are at risk for occult but significant prostate cancer. The ability of multiparametric magnetic resonance imaging/ ultrasound fusion biopsy to detect these occult prostate lesions may make it an effective tool in this challenging scenario.

Materials and Methods.—Between March 2007 and November 2011 all men underwent prostate 3 T endorectal coil magnetic resonance imaging. All concerning lesions were targeted with magnetic resonance imaging/ ultrasound fusion biopsy. In addition, all patients underwent standard 12-core transrectal ultrasound biopsy. Men with 1 or more negative systematic prostate biopsies were included in our cohort.

Results.—Of the 195 men with previous negative biopsies, 73 (37%) were found to have cancer using the magnetic resonance imaging/ultrasound fusion biopsy combined with 12-core transrectal ultrasound biopsy. High grade cancer (Gleason score 8+) was discovered in 21 men (11%), all of whom had disease detected with magnetic resonance imaging/ultrasound fusion biopsy. However, standard transrectal ultrasound biopsy missed 12 of these high grade cancers (55%). Pathological upgrading occurred in 28 men (38.9%) as a result of magnetic resonance imaging/ultrasound fusion targeting vs standard transrectal ultrasound biopsy. The diagnostic yield of combined magnetic resonance imaging/ultrasound fusion platform was unrelated to the number of previous negative biopsies and persisted despite increasing the number of previous biopsy sessions. On multivariate analysis only prostate specific antigen density and magnetic resonance imaging suspicion level remained significant predictors of cancer.

Conclusions.—Multiparametric magnetic resonance imaging with a magnetic resonance imaging/ultrasound fusion biopsy platform is a novel diagnostic tool for detecting prostate cancer and may be ideally suited for

TABLE 2.—Diagnostic Yield Stratified by Standard TRUS vs Targeted MRI/US Fusion Platform

	All Ca	Low Grade (GS 6)	Intermediate Grade (GS 7)	High Grade (GS 8+)
No. either modality detected Ca	73	28	24	21
No. MRI targeting detected Ca (%)	56 (76.7)	16 (57.1)	19 (79.2)	21 (100)
No. US only guidance detected Ca (%)	45 (61.6)	23 (82.1)	12 (50)	10 (47.6)
No. both methods detected Ca (%)	28 (35.9)	11 (39.3)	7 (29.2)	10 (47.6)
No. MRI targeting upgraded risk (%)	28 (38.4)	5 (17.9)	12 (50)	11 (52.3)

patients with negative transrectal ultrasound biopsies in the face of a persistent clinical suspicion for cancer (Table 2).

▶ Scanning with 3 Tesla magnetic resonance imaging (MRI) is emerging as an important means of evaluating men who are at risk for prostate cancer. Fusion of MRI to transrectal ultrasound scan has a lot of appeal as opposed to pure MRI-guided biopsy, which is cumbersome to perform for both the patient and physician. This group has clearly led the way in evaluating fusion. Table 2 illustrates that their modality is capable of detecting many prostate cancers, especially high-grade prostate cancers in men who have had prior negative biopsy results. More experience with their approach at other centers is needed.

G. L. Andriole, Jr, MD

Is Undetectable Prostate-Specific Antigen Always Reliable to Rule Out Prostate Cancer Recurrence After Radical Prostatectomy?

Schriefer P, Steurer S, Huland H, et al (Univ Med Ctr Eppendorf, Hamburg, Germany)
J Clin Oncol 30:e341-e344, 2012

Background.—Prostate-specific antigen (PSA) is a highly sensitive and organ-specific marker that reflects tumor burden and disease activity in patients with prostate cancer (PCa). If PSA levels can be measured after radical prostatectomy (RP), prostatic tissue (tumor) is believed present. If levels are undetectable, the result is considered clear proof of a cure, so the standard follow-up after RP is serial measurements of PSA. However, two patients with undetectable PSA levels were found to have recurrence of their PCa.

Case Reports.—Case 1 Man, 53, was diagnosed with PCa, Gleason 3 (+) 3 in seven of 10 core biopsies. His clinical stage was T2a and PSA level was 15.56 ng/mL, with no sign of metastasis on bone scan or computed tomography (CT) of the abdomen. After RP, surgical margins were negative and no lymph node metastases were found. Five months later the patient complained of pelvic pain although PSA levels remained less than detectable. A lesion at the fifth cervical vertebra and a mass at the left neurovascular bundle were revealed on magnetic resonance imaging (MRI), with CT-guided biopsy showing benign fibromuscular tissue. PCa recurrence being extremely improbable, the mass was viewed as scar tissue. Five months later the patient sought treatment in the emergency department for his poor health, which included fevers, night sweats, tachycardia, hot flushes, and weight loss over the previous 6 weeks. PSA was undetectable but neuron-specific enolase (NSE) level was 40 μg/L and the pelvic lesion showed growth on CT. Prostate origin for the mass was confirmed, and metastases were identified in the liver, lungs, and various bones. The mass progressed despite radiotherapy plus chemotherapy, and the patient died 10 months after the tumor recurrence was diagnosed.

Case 2 Man, 68, had PCa, Gleason 5 + 5 in 10 of 11 cores, clinical stage T2c, and a PSA level of 11.8 ng/mL. RP revealed the tumor had large fractions of necrotic tissue invading the seminal vesicles, diagnosed as a Gleason 5 + 4 pT3b adenocarcinoma. Surgical margins and lymphatic vessel invasion were positive. Two months later the patient developed left-sided hydronephrosis, and a CT scan found a tumorous mass on the bladder's left side that was blocking the left ureteric orifice. Poorly differentiated adenocarcinoma was identified on core biopsy using hematoxylin and eosin staining. Immunohistochemical tests revealed the tissue's prostatic origin and showed a strong possibility for androgen receptor and prostate-specific membrane antigen (PSMA). Repeated measurements of PSA yielded undetectable results, and no distant metastases were found. The tumor was invading vast areas of the pelvis and was not resectable, so an ileal conduit was created for urinary diversion. Radiotherapy produced a reduction in tumor size. The patient's condition was stable 1 year after RP.

Conclusions.—In rare cases it is possible for PCa to recur and metastatic disease to develop even with undetectable PSA levels. In patients who develop symptoms, low or absent PSA levels do not rule out tumor relapse.

▶ This article is a timely reminder that the patient, not his blood test result, matters most. The authors describe patients with symptoms after radical prostatectomy who had undetectable serum prostate-specific antigen (PSA) levels and biopsy-proven disease recurrence. Although these cases are rare, this report highlights the need to listen to the patient and evaluate accordingly. The reasons for a spuriously undetectable PSA in this setting include unrecognized hypogonadism, poorly differentiated tumors, and assay variation.

G. L. Andriole, Jr, MD

Diagnostics/Staging

Image-Guided Prostate Biopsy Using Magnetic Resonance Imaging–Derived Targets: A Systematic Review

Moore CM, Robertson NL, Arsanious N, et al (Univ College London, UK; Croydon Univ Hosp, London, UK; et al)
Eur Urol 63:125-140, 2013

Context.—Technical improvements in prostate magnetic resonance imaging (MRI) have resulted in the use of MRI to target prostate biopsies.

Objective.—To systematically review the literature to compare the accuracy of MRI-targeted biopsy with standard transrectal biopsy in the detection of clinically significant prostate cancer.

Evidence Acquisition.—The PubMed, Embase, and Cochrane databases were searched from inception until December 3, 2011, using the search criteria 'prostate OR prostate cancer' AND 'magnetic resonance imaging OR MRI' AND 'biopsy OR target'. Four reviewers independently assessed 4222 records; 222 records required full review. Fifty unique records (corresponding to 16 discrete patient populations) directly compared an MRI-targeted with a standard transrectal approach.

Evidence Synthesis.—Evidence synthesis was used to address specific questions. Where MRI was applied to all biopsy-naive men, 62% (374 of 599) had MRI abnormalities. When subjected to a targeted biopsy, 66% (248 of 374) had prostate cancer detected. Both targeted and standard biopsy detected clinically significant cancer in 43% (236 or 237 of 555, respectively). Missed clinically significant cancers occurred in 13 men using targeted biopsy and 12 using a standard approach. Targeted biopsy was more efficient. A third fewer men were biopsied overall. Those who had biopsy required a mean of 3.8 targeted cores compared with 12 standard cores. A targeted approach avoided the diagnosis of clinically insignificant cancer in 53 of 555 (10%) of the presenting population.

Conclusions.—MRI-guided biopsy detects clinically significant prostate cancer in an equivalent number of men versus standard biopsy. This is achieved using fewer biopsies in fewer men, with a reduction in the diagnosis of clinically insignificant cancer. Variability in study methodology limits the strength of recommendation that can be made. There is a need for a robust multicentre trial of targeted biopsies.

▶ This is a timely review of the current status of prostate magnetic resonance imaging (MRI) in the evaluation of men who may have prostate cancer. Several centers around the world have reported that MRI enhances the diagnostic accuracy of prostate needle biopsy, particularly for significant tumors. This report describes the information gaps that exist: What is the best MRI methodology? Can MRI predict Gleason score? What is the best means of performing an MRI targeted biopsy? Is MRI-ultrasound fusion necessary and feasible? I suspect that we will answer these questions in the upcoming years and that MRI will have a place in the diagnosis of prostate cancer, its therapy (eg, image-guided ablation), and monitoring men on active surveillance.

G. L. Andriole, Jr, MD

Transition Zone Prostate Cancer: Detection and Localization with 3-T Multiparametric MR Imaging

Hoeks CMA, Hambrock T, Yakar D, et al (Radboud Univ Nijmegen Med Centre, the Netherlands)
Radiology 266:207-217, 2013

Purpose.—To retrospectively compare transition zone (TZ) cancer detection and localization accuracy of 3-T T2-weighted magnetic resonance (MR) imaging with that of multiparametric (MP) MR imaging, with radical prostatectomy specimens as the reference standard.

Materials and Methods.—The informed consent requirement was waived by the institutional review board. Inclusion criteria were radical prostatectomy specimen TZ cancer larger than 0.5 cm^3 and 3-T endorectal presurgery MP MR imaging (T2-weighted imaging, diffusion-weighted [DW] imaging apparent diffusion coefficient [ADC] maps [$b < 1000$ sec/mm^2], and dynamic contrast material–enhanced [DCE] MR imaging). From 197 patients with radical prostatectomy specimens, 28 patients with TZ cancer were included. Thirty-five patients without TZ cancer were randomly selected as a control group. Four radiologists randomly scored T2-weighted and DW ADC images, T2-weighted and DCE MR images, and T2-weighted, DW ADC, and DCE MR images. TZ cancer suspicion was rated on a five-point scale in six TZ regions of interest (ROIs). A score of 4–5 was considered a positive finding. A score of 4 or higher for any ROI containing TZ cancer was considered a positive detection result at the patient level. Generalized estimating equations were used to analyze detection and localization accuracy by using ROI-receiver operating characteristics (ROC) curve analyses for the latter. Gleason grade (GG) 4–5 and GG 2-3 cancers were analyzed separately.

Results.—Detection accuracy did not differ between T2-weighted and MP MR imaging for all TZ cancers (68% vs 66%, $P = .85$), GG 4–5 TZ cancers (79% vs 72%–75%, $P = .13$), and GG 2–3 TZ cancers (66% vs 62%–65%, $P = .47$). MP MR imaging (area under the ROC curve, 0.70–0.77) did not improve T2-weighted imaging localization accuracy (AUC = 0.72) ($P > .05$).

Conclusion.—Use of 3-T MP MR imaging, consisting of T2-weighted imaging, DW imaging ADC maps (b values, 50, 500, and 800 sec/mm^2), and DCE MR imaging may not improve TZ cancer detection and localization accuracy compared with T2-weighted imaging.

▶ One of the important uses of magnetic resonance imaging in detecting prostate cancer is in men with elevated prostate-specific antigen levels whose biopsy of the peripheral zone does not show cancer. Often, if a cancer was missed by the biopsy, it is because the tumor was located in the transition zone of the prostate, which is more anterior and would generally require a targeted biopsy for detection. In this study, the authors show that these tumors are well detected on

T2 imaging, which is widely available, and that there is little added benefit to multiparametric imaging with diffusion-weighted imaging.

G. L. Andriole, Jr, MD

Contemporary Grading for Prostate Cancer: Implications for Patient Care
Brimo F, Montironi R, Egevad L, et al (McGill Univ Health Ctr, Quebec, Canada; Polytechnic Univ of the Marche Region, Ancona, Italy; Karolinska Inst, Stockholm, Sweden; et al)
Eur Urol 63:892-901, 2013

Context.—The Gleason grading system is one of the most powerful predictors of outcome in prostate cancer and a cornerstone in counseling and treating patients. Since its inception, it has undergone several modifications triggered by a change in clinical practice and a better understanding of the cancer's histologic spectrum and variants and their prognostic significance.

Objective.—To provide an overview of the implementation and the impact of the Gleason system as a predictive and prognostic tool in all available treatment modalities, and to compare the original and modified Gleason systems in major pathologic and clinical outcome data sets.

Evidence Acquisition.—A comprehensive nonsystematic Medline search was performed using multiple Medical Subject Headings such as *Gleason, modified, system, outcome, biopsy, prostatectomy, recurrence, prognosis, radiotherapy,* and *focal therapy,* with restriction to the English language and a preference for publications within the last 10 yr. All Gleason grade-related studies in the last 3 yr were reviewed. For studies before this date, we relied on prior culling of the literature for various recent books, chapters, and original articles on this topic.

Evidence Synthesis.—Using the modified grading system resulted in disease upgrading with more cancers assigned a Gleason score ≥7 than in the past. It also resulted in a more homogeneous Gleason score 6, which has an excellent prognosis when the disease is organ confined. The vast majority of studies using both systems showed that Gleason grading of adenocarcinomas on needle biopsies and radical prostatectomies was strongly associated with pathologic stage, status of surgical margins, metastatic disease, biochemical recurrence, and cancer-specific survival, with the modified system outperforming the original one in some large series. A description of the continuous incorporation of this parameter in the clinical decision making for treating prostate cancer using all currently used treatment modalities is presented, and the findings of studies before and after the inception of the modified grading system, if available, are compared. The proposed contemporary grading prognostic categories are 3 + 3, 3 + 4, 4 + 3, 8, and 9−10.

Conclusions.—The Gleason score is one of the most critical predictive factors of prostate cancer regardless of the therapy used. Modernization of the Gleason grading system has resulted in a more accurate grading

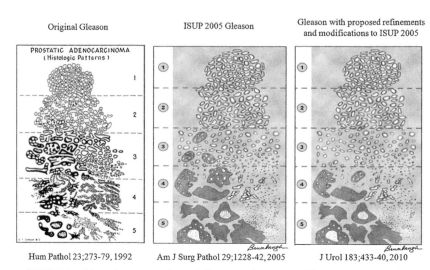

Original Gleason   ISUP 2005 Gleason   Gleason with proposed refinements and modifications to ISUP 2005

Hum Pathol 23;273-79, 1992   Am J Surg Pathol 29;1228-42, 2005   J Urol 183;433-40, 2010

FIGURE 1.—Schematic representations of Gleason grading systems. The most important changes between them are in patterns 3 and 4. In the modified system, most cribriform patterns and also poorly defined glands are included in pattern 4. In the currently used system, all cribriform glands are included as pattern 4. (Reprinted from Brimo F, Montironi R, Egevad L, et al. Contemporary grading for prostate cancer: Implications for patient care. *Eur Urol.* 2013;63:892-901, Copyright 2013, with permission from European Association of Urology.)

system for radical prostatectomy (RP) but has complicated the comparison of data before and after the updating. A better prognostication with the updated Gleason grading system for patients treated with modalities other than surgery can only be postulated at this time because there are limited conflicting data on radiation and no studies on other treatment modalities. Its greatest impact is the uniformly excellent prognosis associated with Gleason score 6 in RPs (Fig 1).

▶ This thoughtful article reviews the contemporary use of the Gleason scoring system to predict outcome of men with prostate cancer. In so doing, it pictorially reviews the series of modification to the original scoring system, as shown in Fig 1. Their proposed regrouping of Gleason scores into 6, 3 + 4, 4 + 3, 8, and 9 to 10 is supported by data from radical prostatectomy outcomes. One wonders how the predictive power of this system will be enhanced, or perhaps supplanted, by genetic classification.

G. L. Andriole, Jr, MD

Primary Cancers Before and After Prostate Cancer Diagnosis

Van Hemelrijck M, Drevin L, Holmberg L, et al (King's College London, UK; Regional Cancer Ctr Uppsala Orebro, Sweden; et al)
Cancer 118:6207-6216, 2012

Background.—The occurrence of multiple cancers may indicate common etiology; and, although some studies have investigated the risk of second primary cancers after prostate cancer (PCa), there are no studies on cancers before PCa.

Methods.—The PCBaSe Sweden database is based on the National Prostate Cancer Register (NPCR), which covers >96% of PCa cases. The authors estimated the prevalence and cumulative incidence of different cancers before and after PCa diagnosis in 72,613 men according to PCa treatment and disease stage in PCBaSe and their matched comparison cohort of men who were free of PCa.

Results.—In total, 6829 men were diagnosed with another primary cancer before their PCa diagnosis, including 138 men at the time of PCa diagnosis and 5230 men were diagnosed after PCa diagnosis. Cancer of the bladder or colon and nonmelanoma of the skin were the 3 most frequently observed cancers before and after PCa diagnosis. At the time of PCa diagnosis, the prevalence of these 3 cancers was 1.94% for bladder cancer, 1.08% for colon cancer, and 1.08% for nonmelanoma skin cancer, compared with 1.30%, 0.96%, and 1.03%, respectively, for the matched comparison cohort. Five years after PCa diagnosis, the difference in incidence proportion between PCa men and their comparison cohort was $7\%_{oo}$ (95% CI, $5.6\%_{oo}$-$8.5\%_{oo}$), $1.3\%_{oo}$ ($0\%_{oo}$-$2.6\%_{oo}$), and $1.6\%_{oo}$ ($0.6\%_{oo}$-$2.6\%_{oo}$) for these 3 cancers, respectively. From a uro-oncologic point of view, it is interesting to note that the prevalence of kidney cancer at the time of PCa diagnosis was 0.42% compared with 0.28% for the matched comparison cohort.

Conclusions.—Approximately 17% of all PCa occurred in combination with another primary cancer (before or after PCa diagnosis). Detection bias probably explains part of this observation, but further investigations are required to assess possible underlying mechanisms.

▶ This is an eye-opening report that quantifies that a large proportion of men with prostate cancer have or are at risk to have other cancers. In some cases, treatment of the other cancers may be more relevant to the patient's outcome. Add to this the association of radiation with the development of bladder cancer, and it becomes clear that those who monitor men with prostate cancer have to be on the lookout for other cancers.

G. L. Andriole, Jr, MD

Natural History/Outcomes

Projecting Prostate Cancer Mortality in the PCPT and REDUCE Chemoprevention Trials

Pinsky PF, Black A, Grubb R, et al (Natl Cancer Inst, Bethesda, MD; Washington Univ, St Louis, MO; et al)
Cancer 119:593-601, 2013

Background.—Two recent chemoprevention trials demonstrated significant reductions in overall prostate cancer incidence. However, a possible increase in high-grade disease has raised concerns that the harms of the drugs, including mortality because of high-grade disease, may outweigh the benefits. The authors attempted to estimate the effect of these drugs on prostate cancer mortality to be able to better evaluate the cost-benefit tradeoff.

Methods.—The authors analyzed prostate cancer incidence in the Prostate Cancer Prevention Trial (PCPT) and Reduction by Dutasteride of Prostate Cancer Events (REDUCE) trial, which evaluated finasteride and the related compound dutasteride, respectively (both vs placebo). They used 13-year prostate cancer survival data from the Prostate, Lung, Colorectal and Ovarian (PLCO) trial to project prostate cancer mortality from incidence patterns; survival rates were applied to incident cancers according to prognostic strata, which were defined by Gleason score, prostate-specific antigen level, and clinical stage. For PCPT, the analysis was performed using both original trial results and previously published adjusted analyses that attempted to account for artifacts related to the drugs' effect on prostate volume.

Results.—For the PCPT trial, the estimated relative risk (RR) for prostate cancer mortality was 1.02 (95% confidence interval [95% CI], 0.85-1.23) using the original trial results and 0.87 (95% CI, 0.72-1.06) and 0.91 (95% CI, 0.76-1.09) based on the adjusted PCPT analyses. For the REDUCE trial, the RR for prostate cancer mortality was 0.93 (95% CI, 0.80-1.08).

Conclusions.—Projecting a mortality outcome of the PCPT and REDUCE trials as an approach to weighing benefits versus harms suggests at most a small increase in prostate cancer mortality in the treatment arms, and possibly a modest decrease.

▶ One of the controversies about the use of 5α reductase inhibitors to reduce the diagnosis of prostate cancer among men undergoing screening is that these agents may possibly induce high-grade tumors, a concern that persists despite ample evidence that various biases, such as a smaller prostate volume at the time of biopsy and enhanced utility of prostate-specific antigen in the treated men, account for the numerical excess of high-grade tumors. This study looks at projected mortality from prostate cancers detected in both Prostate Cancer Prevention Trial (PCPT) and Reduction by Dutasteride of Prostate Cancer Events using survival data from the Prostate, Lung, Colorectal and Ovarian cancer screening trial. This projection suggests that there would be no excess prostate cancer mortality. It is likely that the actual survival data from PCPT will soon be forthcoming.

G. L. Andriole, Jr, MD

Active Surveillance of Very-low-risk Prostate Cancer in the Setting of Active Treatment of Benign Prostatic Hyperplasia With 5α-reductase Inhibitors
Shelton PQ, Ivanowicz AN, Wakeman CM, et al (Carolinas Med Ctr, Charlotte, NC; Levine Cancer Inst, Charlotte, NC)
Urology 81:979-985, 2013

Objective. To review the efficacy of treating benign prostatic hyperplasia and very-low-risk prostate cancer (PCa) in patients receiving active surveillance and 5α-reductase inhibitor (5-ARI; finasteride or dutasteride) treatment.

Materials and Methods.—Eighty-two men with very-low-risk PCa (clinical stage T1c, Gleason score ≤ 6, <3 biopsy cores positive with ≤50% involvement, and prostate-specific antigen density ≤ 0.15 ng/mL/g) and benign prostatic hyperplasia (≥30 cm^3) received active surveillance and were treated with a 5-ARI.

Results.—All 82 men completed 1 year of 5-ARI therapy (n = 79) or underwent early biopsy for cause (n = 3). Restaging biopsies were performed for 76 men (22 underwent a second restaging biopsy and 1 a third restaging biopsy), 4 patients were awaiting biopsy, and 2 were lost to follow-up before the first restaging biopsy. At the first restaging biopsy, of the 76 men, 41 (54%) had no PCa, 16 (21%) continued to have very-low-risk PCa, 15 (20%) had progressed to low-risk PCa (>2 cores positive and Gleason score ≤ 6), and 4 (5%) had progressed to intermediate-risk PCa (Gleason score 7). Of the 76 biopsies, 20 were performed early for cause, with 11 (55%) showing PCa progression. Of the 82 patients, 22 (27%) underwent treatment of PCa.

Conclusion.—Active surveillance of very-low-risk PCa in the setting of 5-ARI therapy for benign prostatic hyperplasia appears to be a safe therapeutic option, because most (57 of 82; 70%) patients maintained very-low-risk PCa or had negative follow-up biopsies during a 3-year follow-up period. Complementary to the Prostate Cancer Prevention Trial, our results indicate that 5-ARI therapy increases prostate-specific antigen sensitivity and can aid the clinician in appropriately targeting biopsies.

▶ The possibility that use of 5α-reductase inhibitors (5ARI) may enhance the efficacy of active surveillance of men with low-risk prostate cancer has been addressed in the REDEEM randomized trial of dutasteride vs placebo and now in a real world series. Both reports show that over 2 to 3 years, 5ARI are safe, seem to reduce benign prostatic hyperplasia—related complications, seem to enhance the chance of a negative follow-up biopsy (since these agents may well shrink low grade tumors), and improve ability of prostate-specific antigen (by using rise from the posttreatment nadir) to identify aggressive prostate cancer.

G. L. Andriole, Jr, MD

Evidence of Perineural Invasion on Prostate Biopsy Specimen and Survival After Radical Prostatectomy

Delancey JO, Wood DP Jr, He C, et al (Univ of Michigan, Ann Arbor; VA Ann Arbor Healthcare System, MI)
Urology 81:354-357, 2013

Objective.—To better understand relationships between perineural invasion (PNI) and radical prostatectomy outcomes, we examined whether PNI was independently associated with adverse pathologic features and worse survival outcomes after radical prostatectomy.

Methods.—PNI is a routinely reported pathologic parameter for prostate biopsy specimens. We identified 3226 patients undergoing radical prostatectomy for clinically localized prostate cancer at our institution between 1994 and 2010. We used multivariable logistic regression models to examine whether PNI was independently associated with extraprostatic extension, seminal vesicle invasion, and surgical margin status. We used Kaplan-Meier methods and the log-rank test to assess disease-free, prostate cancer-specific, and overall survival according to PNI status. Cox proportional hazards modeling was used to evaluate relationships between PNI and survival outcomes.

Results.—PNI was identified in the prostate biopsy specimen in 20% of patients who underwent radical prostatectomy. Patients with PNI were more likely to have adverse pathologic features, including extraprostatic extension, seminal vesicle invasion, and positive surgical margins. Patients with PNI had shorter disease-free, cancer-specific, and overall survival (all log-rank $P < .001$). After adjustment for adverse pathologic features at radical prostatectomy, PNI was independently associated with disease-free survival (adjusted hazard ratio, 1.45; 95% confidence interval, 1.09-1.92) and overall survival (hazard ratio, 1.57; 95% confidence interval, 1.13-2.18).

Conclusion.—PNI was independently associated with adverse pathologic features and worse survival outcomes after radical prostatectomy. For these reasons, PNI on prostate biopsy specimens should be considered in prostate cancer treatment decision making and clinical care (Fig).

▶ This well-performed analysis confirms the perineural invasion detected on needle biopsy is an adverse finding, as shown in Fig. Practitioners should consider this information when counseling men with newly diagnosed prostate cancer.

G. L. Andriole, Jr, MD

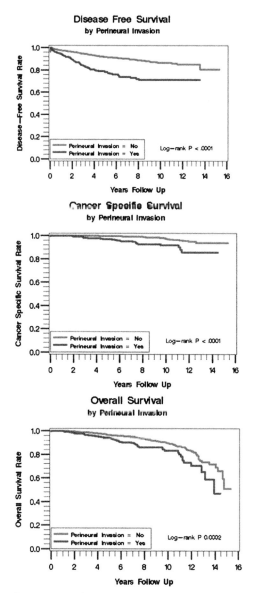

FIGURE.—Disease-free, cancer-specific, and overall survival after radical prostatectomy are shown by perineural invasion (PNI) status on the prostate biopsy specimen. Patients without PNI on their prostate biopsy specimen had significantly longer disease-free, cancer-specific, and overall survival (all log-rank *P* < .001) than patients with evidence of PNI. After adjustment for adverse pathologic features at radical prostatectomy, PNI was independently associated with disease-free survival (adjusted hazard ratio, 1.45; 95% confidence interval, 1.09-1.92) and overall survival (hazard ratio, 1.57; 95% confidence interval, 1.13-2.18) but not with cancer-specific survival. (Color version available online.) (Reprinted from Delancey JO, Wood DP Jr, He C, et al. Evidence of perineural invasion on prostate biopsy specimen and survival after radical prostatectomy. *Urology.* 2013;81:354-357, Copyright 2013, with permission from Elsevier.)

Orgasm-Associated Incontinence (Climacturia) after Bladder Neck-Sparing Radical Prostatectomy: Clinical and Video-Urodynamic Evaluation

Manassero F, Di Paola G, Paperini D, et al (Univ of Pisa, Italy; et al)
J Sex Med 9:2150-2156, 2012

Introduction.—Orgasm-Associated Incontinence (OAI) or climacturia has been observed in male patients maintaining sexual potency after radical prostatectomy and cystectomy.

Aim.—We investigated the incidence and video-urodynamic aspects of this event in continent and potent patients after bladder neck-sparing (BNS) radical prostatectomy (RP).

Main Outcome Measure.—Comparing functional and morphological aspects between climacturic and non-climacturic patients to identify a possible explanation of this unusual kind of leakage that could seriously impact the sexual life after surgery.

Methods.—In a pool of 84 men, potent and continent at least 1 year after BNS RP, 24 (28.6%) reported climacturia and 7 agreed to undergo video-urodynamic evaluation (group 1), which was performed also in 5 controls (group 2). Those 12 men were also evaluated with 24-hour pad test, 5-item International Index of Erectile Function and International Prostate Symptom Score questionnaires.

Results.—Functional urethral length (FUL) was significantly lower in the climacturia group ($P = 0.02$) and time to continence recovery was significantly longer ($P = 0.05$). No other significant differences were found between the two groups. The radiological appearance of the vesicourethral junction at voiding cystourethrography was similar.

Conclusions.—To the best of our knowledge, this is the first functional and morphological evaluation of climacturia after RP. In our experience, this event is indirectly associated with a reduced FUL in the sphincter area, although both patients and controls were continent during daily activities. BNS technique seems to reduce time to continence recovery, although climacturic patients need longer time than control patients. Since in our series no rigidity of the vesicourethral anastomosis was radiographically evident, we believe that differences in FUL could explain OAI. Anatomical difference in membranous urethra length could explain the occurrence of this symptom in patients treated with the same surgical technique.

▶ This population of men was investigated for the presence of climacturia, defined as loss of urine with sexual activity and/or orgasm. Climacturia typically occurs in men who are post radical prostatectomy. This problem may remain in some men even after functional urinary continence is restored.

The prevalence of climacturia in this group (minimum 1 year out) was about 30%, in line with other published data and indicative of a very common but little discussed problem. Climacturia may be of little clinical consequence, particularly in low-volume settings, but it can be psychologically distressing and may make certain sexual activities unacceptably unhygienic for some couples.

Unfortunately, just 12 patients were included in this study so it is difficult to know how universal decreased urethral length is in patients with climacturia. Further work on this little studied problem may provide clues on how to best manage these patients.

A. W. Shindel, MD

Treatment Comparison

Long-Term Functional Outcomes after Treatment for Localized Prostate Cancer

Resnick MJ, Koyama T, Fan K-II, et al (Vanderbilt Univ, Nashville, TN; et al)
N Engl J Med 368:436-445, 2013

Background.—The purpose of this analysis was to compare long-term urinary, bowel, and sexual function after radical prostatectomy or external-beam radiation therapy.

Methods.—The Prostate Cancer Outcomes Study (PCOS) enrolled 3533 men in whom prostate cancer had been diagnosed in 1994 or 1995. The current cohort comprised 1655 men in whom localized prostate cancer had been diagnosed between the ages of 55 and 74 years and who had undergone either surgery (1164 men) or radiotherapy (491 men). Functional status was assessed at baseline and at 2, 5, and 15 years after diagnosis. We used multivariable propensity scoring to compare functional outcomes according to treatment.

Results.—Patients undergoing prostatectomy were more likely to have urinary incontinence than were those undergoing radiotherapy at 2 years (odds ratio, 6.22; 95% confidence interval [CI], 1.92 to 20.29) and 5 years (odds ratio, 5.10, 95% CI, 2.29 to 11.36). However, no significant between-group difference in the odds of urinary incontinence was noted at 15 years. Similarly, although patients undergoing prostatectomy were more likely to have erectile dysfunction at 2 years (odds ratio, 3.46; 95% CI, 1.93 to 6.17) and 5 years (odds ratio, 1.96; 95% CI, 1.05 to 3.63), no significant between-group difference was noted at 15 years. Patients undergoing prostatectomy were less likely to have bowel urgency at 2 years (odds ratio, 0.39; 95% CI, 0.22 to 0.68) and 5 years (odds ratio, 0.47; 95% CI, 0.26 to 0.84), again with no significant between-group difference in the odds of bowel urgency at 15 years.

Conclusions.—At 15 years, no significant relative differences in disease-specific functional outcomes were observed among men undergoing prostatectomy or radiotherapy. Nonetheless, men treated for localized prostate cancer commonly had declines in all functional domains during 15 years of follow-up.

▶ This report examines long-term functional outcomes of men after definitive treatment for prostate cancer with external beam radiation or radical prostatectomy. Subjects were recruited in the mid-1990s from 6 centers around the United States. As detailed in the abstract, the rate of bowel symptoms was higher in the radiation group at 2 and 5 years, but the difference was not statistically significant at 15 years. Similarly, the rate of urinary incontinence and erectile dysfunction was higher in the surgery group at the 2- and 5-year time points, but the rate was not statistically significant at 15-year follow-up. It is worth noting that the rates of erectile dysfunction (ED) at the 15-year time point for the surgery and radiation therapy groups were 87% and 94%, respectively; in other words, most men had ED at that time point.

This study likely represents regression to the mean at the 15-year time point; steady accumulation of comorbidities will likely blur differences in functional outcomes between groups as the treatment event becomes more remote. Indeed, it is not surprising that both treatment groups had declines in all 3 domains at 15-year follow-up; a control group of men without prostate cancer or prostate cancer treatment would likely have the same finding.

Urologists are likely to take issue with the higher rate of ED and incontinence in the surgical treatment arm. The data are what they are, but it is important to recognize that the radiation therapy sample was much smaller than the prosta-tectomy sample; this may skew results to some extent. Selection of the binary endpoints (ED or no ED, incontinence or no incontinence) and use of some-what arbitrary cut-offs to do so may have also introduced some bias.

A principle and important limitation is that baseline sexual, urinary, and bowel functions were obtained retrospectively 6 months after treatment. It is very likely that some men, struggling with the early phase of recovery from cancer treatment, overestimated their pretreatment level of function, although the authors of this study provide a citation to argue that this effect is minimal.

This represents one of the longest prospective observational studies of prostate cancer treatment in the United States. Urologists should read this article carefully and know how to address its findings with patients. Urologists should also counsel patients that the only interventions shown to reliably reverse/prevent/slow down the progression of ED in any setting (prostate cancer or no) is a combination of healthy diet, maintenance of normal body weight/waist circum-ference, and routine physical activity.

A. W. Shindel, MD

Long-Term Functional Outcomes after Treatment for Localized Prostate Cancer
Resnick MJ, Koyama T, Fan K-H, et al (Vanderbilt Univ, Nashville, TN; et al)
N Engl J Med 368:436-445, 2013

Background.—The purpose of this analysis was to compare long-term urinary, bowel, and sexual function after radical prostatectomy or external-beam radiation therapy.

Methods.—The Prostate Cancer Outcomes Study (PCOS) enrolled 3533 men in whom prostate cancer had been diagnosed in 1994 or 1995. The current cohort comprised 1655 men in whom localized prostate cancer had been diagnosed between the ages of 55 and 74 years and who had under-gone either surgery (1164 men) or radiotherapy (491 men). Functional

TABLE 2.—Survey Responses on Selected Items Regarding Urinary, Bowel, and Sexual Function*

Outcome	Prostatectomy *percent*	Radiotherapy	Adjusted Odds Ratio (95% CI)[†]
Urinary incontinence			
No control or frequent urinary leakage			
2 yr	9.6	3.2	6.22 (1.92–20.29)
5 yr	13.4	4.4	5.10 (2.29–11.36)
15 yr	18.3	9.4	2.34 (0.88–6.23)
Bothered by dripping or leaking urine[‡]			
2 yr	10.6	2.4	5.86 (1.93–17.64)
5 yr	12.9	2.9	7.66 (2.97–19.89)
15 yr	17.1	18.4	0.87 (0.41–1.80)
Sexual function			
Erection insufficient for intercourse			
2 yr	78.8	60.8	3.46 (1.93–6.17)
5 yr	75.7	71.9	1.96 (1.05–3.63)
15 yr	87.0	93.9	0.38 (0.12–1.22)
Bothered by sexual dysfunction[‡]			
2 yr	55.5	48.2	1.19 (0.77–1.86)
5 yr	46.7	39.7	1.48 (0.92–2.39)
15 yr	43.5	37.7	1.33 (0.58–3.03)
Bowel function			
Bowel urgency			
2 yr	13.6	34.0	0.39 (0.22–0.68)
5 yr	16.3	31.3	0.47 (0.26–0.84)
15 yr	21.9	35.8	0.98 (0.45–2.14)
Bothered by frequent bowel movements, pain, or urgency[‡]			
2 yr	2.9	7.9	0.37 (0.14–0.96)
5 yr	4.4	5.8	0.93 (0.27–3.22)
15 yr	5.2	16.0	0.29 (0.11–0.78)

*All percentages were adjusted for sampling weight.
[†]Odds ratios are for the prostatectomy group as compared with the radiotherapy group. Odds ratios have been adjusted for registry, age, baseline function, race or ethnic group, tumor grade, number of coexisting illnesses, education level, and propensity score.
[‡]Survey respondents described being bothered as either a "moderate problem" or "big problem."

status was assessed at baseline and at 2, 5, and 15 years after diagnosis. We used multivariable propensity scoring to compare functional outcomes according to treatment.

Results.—Patients undergoing prostatectomy were more likely to have urinary incontinence than were those undergoing radiotherapy at 2 years (odds ratio, 6.22; 95% confidence interval [CI], 1.92 to 20.29) and 5 years (odds ratio, 5.10; 95% CI, 2.29 to 11.36). However, no significant between-group difference in the odds of urinary incontinence was noted at 15 years. Similarly, although patients undergoing prostatectomy were more likely to have erectile dysfunction at 2 years (odds ratio, 3.46; 95% CI, 1.93 to 6.17) and 5 years (odds ratio, 1.96; 95% CI, 1.05 to 3.63), no significant between-group difference was noted at 15 years. Patients undergoing prostatectomy were less likely to have bowel urgency at 2 years (odds ratio, 0.39; 95% CI, 0.22 to 0.68) and 5 years (odds ratio, 0.47; 95% CI, 0.26 to 0.84), again with no significant between-group difference in the odds of bowel urgency at 15 years.

Conclusions.—At 15 years, no significant relative differences in disease-specific functional outcomes were observed among men undergoing prostatectomy or radiotherapy. Nonetheless, men treated for localized prostate cancer commonly had declines in all functional domains during 15 years of follow-up. (Funded by the National Cancer Institute.) (Table 2).

▶ This trial followed quality of life in men with localized prostate cancer who selected either surgery or radiation therapy. It shows the expected declines in urinary, bowel, and sexual function induced by both treatments. It is interesting that, although there were certain differences in the short term (Table 2), by 15 years there was essentially no difference.

G. L. Andriole, Jr, MD

Watchful Waiting/Outcomes

Strengthening evidence for active surveillance for prostate cancer
Klotz L (Univ of Toronto, Ontario, Canada)
Eur Urol 63:108-110, 2013

Background.—Clinicians are happy to embrace new diagnostic tools that allow one to make a diagnosis early on in the course of diseases that benefit from early intervention. However, in some cases the diagnosis of disease is made in patients who would never have been diagnosed before death without such an advanced screening device. The results include overdiagnosis and overtreatment. This is a situation facing clinicians with respect to prostate cancer (PCa), but potentially could also occur with diabetes, chronic renal failure, hypertension, and cancers of the breast, lung, and thyroid, as well as other disorders. The answers to such problems include restricting screening efforts to those persons at higher risk and reducing the burden of therapy by avoiding unneeded treatment. Active surveillance (AS) has also been used in PCa as a result of studies such as the Göteborg randomized, population-based, prostate cancer screening trials.

Relevant Findings.—The results of the Göteborg trial are consistent with other phase 2 studies of AS already published. Among a uniformly screened population of men diagnosed with PCa, nearly 50% can be managed safely with AS for intermediate periods. About a third of patients were eventually treated. Many radical prostatectomy studies have found that of men who are at low risk for disease after transrectal ultrasound (TRUS)? guided systematic biopsy, about 25% to 30% will be harboring high-grade disease. This percentage of men who are eventually treated after a period of surveillance is markedly consistent between studies.

Recommendations.—Identifying men at low risk who harbor higher grade disease at the time of diagnosis or shortly thereafter is ideal and would permit earlier treatment of those affected as well as reassurance for the men who remain under AS. Multiparametric magnetic resonance imaging (MRI) may be able to identify those who have large anterior cancers early in the disease course. The Göteborg trial shows that it is necessary to treat 12 men for each PCa mortality avoided and supports the use of AS for patients at low risk for disease.

Conclusions.—The benefits of treatment in PCa tend to accrue to patients at intermediate or high risk for disease rather than to those at low risk for disease. Progression of the prostate-specific antigen (PSA) levels is more appropriate as an indicator of the need for additional biopsies rather than as a trigger for intervention. The challenge remains to identify low-risk patients who harbor occult aggressive disease and would benefit from early treatment. Predictive biomarkers are being actively sought to help in this endeavor, but none of those investigated so far have proved sufficiently reliable to be used in clinical practice.

▶ There is no more important issue in prostate cancer than identifying the appropriate selection of men for active surveillance and defining the appropriate monitoring strategy (eg, prostate-specific antigen, prostate cancer antigen-3, MRI, repeat random, or targeted biopsies, and use of genetic markers) for such men. This article presents a nice overview of the current state of the art in this evolving area. It is clear that more men should undergo surveillance, but how best to do it remains elusive at the moment.

G. L. Andriole, Jr, MD

Validation of a Cell-Cycle Progression Gene Panel to Improve Risk Stratification in a Contemporary Prostatectomy Cohort

Cooperberg MR, Simko JP, Cowan JE, et al (Univ of California, San Francisco; et al)
J Clin Oncol 31:1428-1434, 2013

Purpose.—We aimed to validate a previously described genetic risk score, denoted the cell-cycle progression (CCP) score, in predicting contemporary radical prostatectomy (RP) outcomes.

Methods.—RNA was quantified from paraffin-embedded RP specimens. The CCP score was calculated as average expression of 31 CCP genes, normalized to 15 housekeeper genes. Recurrence was defined as two prostate-specific antigen levels ≥ 0.2 ng/mL or any salvage treatment. Associations between CCP score and recurrence were examined, with adjustment for clinical and pathologic variables using Cox proportional hazards regression and partial likelihood ratio tests. The CCP score was assessed for independent prognostic utility beyond a standard postoperative risk assessment (Cancer of the Prostate Risk Assessment post-Surgical [CAPRA-S] score), and a score combining CAPRA-S and CCP was validated.

Results.—Eighty-two (19.9%) of 413 men experienced recurrence. The hazard ratio (HR) for each unit increase in CCP score (range, -1.62 to 2.16) was 2.1 (95% CI, 1.6 to 2.9); with adjustment for CAPRA-S, the HR was 1.7 (95% CI, 1.3 to 2.4). The score was able to substratify patients with low clinical risk as defined by CAPRA-S ≤ 2 (HR, 2.3; 95% CI, 1.4 to

3.7). Combining the CCP and CAPRA-S improved the concordance index for both the overall cohort and low-risk subset; the combined CAPRA-S + CCP score consistently predicted outcomes across the range of clinical risk. This combined score outperformed both individual scores on decision curve analysis.

Conclusion.—The CCP score was validated to have significant prognostic accuracy after controlling for all available clinical and pathologic data. The score may improve accuracy of risk stratification for men with clinically localized prostate cancer, including those with low-risk disease.

▶ We may be entering an era of "personalized" medicine by using patient and tumor-specific genetics to predict outcomes and response to treatment. In this study, the authors show that use of a panel of genetic markers from the cell cycle progression pathway can significantly alter the prediction of outcomes for men with localized prostate cancer in comparison with the use of clinical variables alone. This is illustrated in Fig 2B of the original article, where the addition of the genetic information discloses that some patients considered to have low risk for progression, using clinical variables, actually harbor more aggressive tumors. This information should go a long way to informing decisions about active surveillance or aggressive therapy.

G. L. Andriole, Jr, MD

Radical Prostatectomy Outcomes

Radical Prostatectomy versus Observation for Localized Prostate Cancer
Wilt TJ, for the Prostate Cancer Intervention versus Observation Trial (PIVOT) Study Group (Univ of Minnesota School of Medicine, Minneapolis; et al)
N Engl J Med 367:203-213, 2012

Background.—The effectiveness of surgery versus observation for men with localized prostate cancer detected by means of prostate-specific antigen (PSA) testing is not known.

Methods.—From November 1994 through January 2002, we randomly assigned 731 men with localized prostate cancer (mean age, 67 years; median PSA value, 7.8 ng per milliliter) to radical prostatectomy or observation and followed them through January 2010. The primary outcome was all-cause mortality; the secondary outcome was prostate-cancer mortality.

Results.—During the median follow-up of 10.0 years, 171 of 364 men (47.0%) assigned to radical prostatectomy died, as compared with 183 of 367 (49.9%) assigned to observation (hazard ratio, 0.88; 95% confidence interval [CI], 0.71 to 1.08; $P = 0.22$; absolute risk reduction, 2.9 percentage points). Among men assigned to radical prostatectomy, 21 (5.8%) died from prostate cancer or treatment, as compared with 31 men (8.4%) assigned to observation (hazard ratio, 0.63; 95% CI, 0.36 to 1.09; $P = 0.09$; absolute risk reduction, 2.6 percentage points). The effect of treatment on all-cause and prostate-cancer mortality did not differ according to age, race, coexisting conditions, self-reported performance status, or histologic features of the

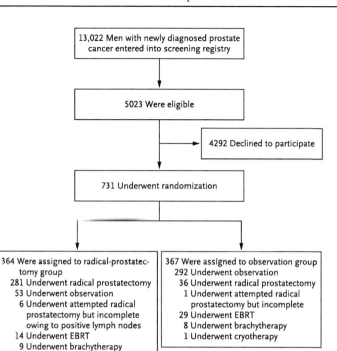

FIGURE 1.—Study enrollment and treatment. Of a total of 13,022 men who were screened for participation, 5023 were eligible for enrollment; of these, 731 were randomly assigned to radical prostatectomy or observation. Of the 364 men in the radical-prostatectomy group, 287 underwent attempted surgery, as did 37 of the 367 men in the observation group. EBRT denotes external-beam radiotherapy. (Reprinted from Wilt TJ, for the Prostate Cancer Intervention versus Observation Trial (PIVOT) Study Group. Radical prostatectomy versus observation for localized prostate cancer. *N Engl J Med.* 2012;367:203-213, © 2012, Massachusetts Medical Society.)

tumor. Radical prostatectomy was associated with reduced all-cause mortality among men with a PSA value greater than 10 ng per milliliter ($P = 0.04$ for interaction) and possibly among those with intermediate-risk or high-risk tumors ($P = 0.07$ for interaction). Adverse events within 30 days after surgery occurred in 21.4% of men, including one death.

Conclusions.—Among men with localized prostate cancer detected during the early era of PSA testing, radical prostatectomy did not significantly reduce all-cause or prostate-cancer mortality, as compared with observation, through at least 12 years of follow-up. Absolute differences were less than 3 percentage points. (Funded by the Department of Veterans Affairs Cooperative Studies Program and others; PIVOT ClinicalTrials. gov number, NCT00007644.) (Fig 1).

▶ Publication of the long awaited Prostate Cancer Intervention versus Observation Trial has unfortunately not put to bed the radical prostatectomy debate. Although the study did not show a survival advantage for radical prostatectomy, if one delves deeper into the data, the results are consistent with surgery benefiting patients. The study found that surgery was favored with a *P* value that approached significance (*P* = .09) (Fig 1). This is despite the fact that only 731 of the planned 2000 patients were enrolled and that at 10 years follow-up, 50% of the patients had died of other causes. In addition, metastasis-free survival clearly favored the surgery group (Supplemental Fig 1), and prostate cancer survival clearly favored surgery in the high-risk patients (Supplemental Fig 3 in the original article). There was absolutely no benefit to surgery in low-risk disease.

I believe that these results are consistent with my thinking about the disease. First, patients with a life expectancy of less than 10 years are unlikely to benefit from surgery. Second, patients with indolent disease are unlikely to benefit from surgery. However, the opposite is probably true too, that patients with longer life expectancy and more aggressive disease are likely to benefit. The finding that metastasis-free survival is improved leads me to believe that with longer follow-up, the benefit of surgery will become more pronounced, particularly in the high-risk patients who are at risk for actually developing metastatic disease.

A. S. Kibel, MD

Effects of Screening on Radical Prostatectomy Efficacy: The Prostate Cancer Intervention Versus Observation Trial

Xia J, Gulati R, Au M, et al (Fred Hutchinson Cancer Res Ctr, Seattle, WA; Univ of Hawaii Cancer Ctr, Honolulu; et al)
J Natl Cancer Inst 105:546-550, 2013

Background.—The Scandinavian Prostate Cancer Group Study Number 4 (SPCG-4) trial showed that radical prostatectomy (RP) reduced prostate cancer deaths with an absolute mortality difference (AMD) between the RP and watchful waiting arms of 6.1% (95% confidence interval [CI] = 0.2% to 12.0%) after 15 years. In the United States, the Prostate Cancer Intervention Versus Observation Trial (PIVOT) produced an AMD of 3% (95% CI = −1.1% to 6.5%) after 12 years. It is not known whether a higher frequency of screen detection in PIVOT explains the lower AMD.

Methods.—We assumed the SPCG-4 trial represents RP efficacy and prostate cancer survival in an unscreened population. Given the fraction of screen-detected prostate cancers in PIVOT, we adjusted prostate cancer survival using published estimates of overdiagnosis and lead time to project the effect of screen detection on disease-specific deaths.

Results.—On the basis of published estimates, we assumed that 32% of screen-detected cancers were overdiagnosed and a mean lead time among non-overdiagnosed cancers of 7.7 years. When we adjusted prostate cancer survival for the 76% of case patients in PIVOT who were screen detected, we projected that the AMD after 12 years would be 2.0% (95% CI = −1.6% to 5.6%) based on variation in published estimates of overdiagnosis and mean lead time in the United States.

Conclusions.—If RP efficacy and prostate cancer survival in the absence of screening are similar to that in the SPCG-4 trial, then overdiagnosis and lead time largely explain the lower AMD in PIVOT. If these artifacts of screening are the correct explanation, then there is a subset of case subjects that should not be treated with RP, and identifying this subset should lead to a clearer understanding of the benefit of RP in the remaining cases.

▶ The Prostate Cancer Intervention Versus Observation Trial (PIVOT) suggested that there was no overall benefit from radical prostatectomy for men with screen-detected cancer, a result that differed from that of the Scandinavian trial of radical prostatectomy that showed a benefit from radical prostatectomy for men younger than 65 who had clinically detected cancer. This analysis shows that a reason for the lack of efficacy of radical prostatectomy in PIVOT is likely to be screening-induced overdiagnosis. This makes sense, as men in PIVOT who had higher prostate-specific antigen levels (> 10) and higher Gleason score (> 6) showed a tendency to benefit from radical prostatectomy. These considerations support the wider institution of active surveilllance for men with low-risk screen-detected cancers.

G. L. Andriole, Jr, MD

The Relationships Between Preoperative Sexual Desire and Quality of Life Following Radical Prostatectomy: A 5-Year Follow-Up Study
Namiki S, Ishidoya S, Nakagawa H, et al (Tohoku Univ Graduate School of Medicine, Sendai, Japan; et al)
J Sex Med 9:2448-2456, 2012

Introduction.—There were few studies about the relationship between sexual desire (SD) and radical prostatectomy (RP).

Aims.— We assessed the relationships between RP and quality of life (QOL) according to the preoperative SD.

Main Outcome Measure.—General QOL was measured with Short Form 36. Sexual function and bother were measured with the University of California, Los Angeles Prostate Cancer Index (PCI). Changes of postoperative SD were also evaluated using PCI.

Methods.—We analyzed data from 285 men who underwent RP and were prospectively enrolled into a longitudinal cohort study. Patients were divided into two groups according to whether they had SD at baseline, which is addressed in the PCI questionnaire: a low SD (LSD) group and a high SD (HSD) group. The assessments were completed before treatment and 3, 6, 12, 24, and 60 months after RP.

Results.—Of the 244 men, 52% had high or a fair level of SD before RP, whereas 48% reported that the level of their SD was low. The HSD group reported better sexual function and sexual bother scores than the LSD group at baseline (both *P* < 0.001). Fifty-one percent of the HSD group reported that SD at 3 months was poor or very poor, which did not return to the preoperative level at all postoperative time points. Nearly 20% of the LSD group regained higher SD after RP than the baseline level. The HSD group showed worse sexual bother scores than the baseline throughout the postoperative follow-up ($P < 0.001$). However, the LSD group demonstrated equivalent sexual bother scores after RP compared with the baseline.

Conclusions.—RP adversely affected SD as well as sexual function and sexual bother. The patients who had HSD experienced greater distress concerning their sexual dysfunction postoperatively than those with LSD.

▶ This study examines the role of sexual desire in predicting sexual function and bother after radical prostatectomy in a prospective cohort of Japanese men. Based on the University of California Los Angeles prostate cancer index, it was determined that men with "low" sexual desire at baseline had minimal change in both sexual bother and function during follow-up; indeed, some patients had enhancement of sexual desire postsurgery. In contrast, there was a steep decline in sexual function and increase in sexual bother in men with high sexual desire at baseline; these changes persisted at all follow-up time points. This is logical in that men with less desire for sex may be less bothered by resulting erectile dysfunction and other sexual problems after prostatectomy; in essence, they perhaps have "less to lose." Importantly, there was essentially no difference in physical and mental health scores between the 2 groups.

What should be done with these data? In my opinion, it is important to assess not just baseline erectile function but also sexual desire in men contemplating radical pelvic surgery. This may help to better tailor counseling on expected outcomes after operation. If present, potential etiologies for distressing absence of sexual desire should be addressed. Patients should also be counseled that sexual desire may decline after radical prostatectomy; whether this is a secondary effect related to erectile dysfunction or other sexual problems is unclear at this time.

A. W. Shindel, MD

Androgen Deprivation

Intermittent Androgen Suppression for Rising PSA Level after Radiotherapy
Crook JM, O'Callaghan CJ, Duncan G, et al (British Columbia Cancer Agency, Kelowna, Canada; Queen's Univ, Kingston, Ontario, Canada; et al)
N Engl J Med 367:895-903, 2012

Background.—Intermittent androgen deprivation for prostate-specific antigen (PSA) elevation after radiotherapy may improve quality of life and delay hormone resistance. We assessed overall survival with intermittent versus continuous androgen deprivation in a noninferiority randomized trial.

Methods.—We enrolled patients with a PSA level greater than 3 ng per milliliter more than 1 year after primary or salvage radiotherapy for localized prostate cancer. Intermittent treatment was provided in 8-month cycles, with nontreatment periods determined according to the PSA level. The primary end point was overall survival. Secondary end points included quality of life, time to castration-resistant disease, and duration of nontreatment intervals.

Results.—Of 1386 enrolled patients, 690 were randomly assigned to intermittent therapy and 696 to continuous therapy. Median follow-up was 6.9 years. There were no significant between-group differences in adverse events. In the intermittent-therapy group, full testosterone recovery occurred in 35% of patients, and testosterone recovery to the trial-entry threshold occurred in 79%. Intermittent therapy provided potential benefits with respect to physical function, fatigue, urinary problems, hot flashes, libido, and erectile function. There were 268 deaths in the intermittent-therapy group and 256 in the continuous-therapy group. Median overall survival was 8.8 years in the intermittent-therapy group versus 9.1 years in the continuous-therapy group (hazard ratio for death, 1.02; 95% confidence interval, 0.86 to 1.21). The estimated 7-year cumulative rates of disease-related death were 18% and 15% in the two groups, respectively ($P = 0.24$).

Conclusions.—Intermittent androgen deprivation was noninferior to continuous therapy with respect to overall survival. Some quality-of-life factors improved with intermittent therapy. (Funded by the Canadian Cancer Society Research Institute and others; ClinicalTrials.gov number, NCT00003653.)

▶ This noninferiority trial demonstrated that intermittent androgen deprivation (ADT) after primary or salvage radiotherapy for localized prostate cancer. Patients were placed on continuous or on intermittent ADT. Intermittent ADT consisted of ADT for 8 months. The ADT was then stopped and only restarted for a prostate-specific antigen (PSA) level of 10 ng/mL. The authors demonstrate equivalent survival in both arms (Fig 1 in the original article). Interestingly, the prostate cancer mortality was higher in the intermittent arm, whereas other causes of death were higher in the continuous arm. Although not statistically significant, these results are consistent with the concept that ADT is not without side effects and is actually associated with significant morbidity and mortality. Because the goal of intermittent therapy is to improve quality of life, it is important to note that although quality of life was better in the intermittent arm, but was not as dramatic as would have been expected, with only a slight improvement.

These results along with other randomized trials have demonstrated that intermittent ADT should not be reserved for the rare patient but should be central in our management of patients with advanced disease, particularly those with PSA recurrences and who have exhausted local therapeutic options. Importantly, it should be done as part of a protocol. Set a PSA level that will result in reinitiating androgen ablation and then stick to it. Also decide on the parameters that will lead to starting continuous therapy.

A. S. Kibel, MD

Advanced Disease

Androgen deprivation therapy before radical prostatectomy is associated with poorer postoperative erectile function outcomes

Mazzola CR, Deveci S, Heck M, et al (Memorial Sloan-Kettering Cancer Ctr, NY)

BJU Int 110:112-116, 2012

Objective.—To define the impact of androgen deprivation therapy (ADT), undergone before radical prostatectomy (RP), on erectile function (EF) recovery.

Material and Methods.—A total of 38 consecutive patients presenting to a sexual medicine clinic after undergoing RP who had received ADT before RP (ADT+ group) were compared with a contemporary, age and comorbidity-matched cohort of 94 patients who did not receive ADT (ADT− group) before undergoing RP.

Medical records were reviewed for demographics, comorbidity profiles and duration of ADT exposure.

All the patients underwent Doppler penile ultrasonography within 6 months of RP and were administered the International Index of Erectile Function (IIEF) questionnaire.

All the patients underwent evaluation of EF recovery. We analysed the incidence of venous leak (VL), mean IIEF EF domain score and proportion of men with EF domain scores ≥ 24 at 18 months after RP.

Results.—The mean age, comorbidity profiles, median Gleason score, median pretreatment PSA level, and mean time to evaluation after RP were similar between the two groups.

The median duration of ADT exposure in the ADT+ group was 3 months.

The incidence of VL within 6 months of surgery was 60% for the ADT+ and 20% for the ADT− group ($P < 0.001$). Likewise, the IIEF EF domain scores and proportion of men with EF domain scores ≥ 24 at 18 months were significantly lower in the ADT+ group, even when controlled for nerve-sparing status.

Conclusion.—Our data suggest that preoperative use of ADT adversely impacts EF outcomes and should therefore be avoided in the absence of robust data suggesting any oncological benefit.

Study Type.—Therapy (case series).

Level of Evidence.—4.

What's known on the subject? and What does the study add?

Erectile dysfunction is a recognized complication of radical prostatectomy. Androgen deprivation therapy adversely impacts sexual function.

Our study shows that the preoperative use of androgen deprivation therapy significantly reduces erectile function recovery after radical prostatectomy. The underneath pathophysiological mechanisms for this to occur are reviewed.

▶ It is not controversial that hormone ablation via leutinizing hormone-releasing hormone agonist or castration exerts a negative effect on erectile function in men. Existing evidence suggests that androgen ablation leads to increased fibrosis, possibly adipose tissue buildup, and predisposition to venous-leak erectile dysfunction in men. Because all other management options for prostate cancer run the same risk, it can be somewhat difficult to parse out the specific treatment that is responsible for a given man's erectile dysfunction after prostate cancer treatment.

This small case-control study from a busy sexual rehabilitation practice investigates the effect of presurgical androgen deprivation therapy (ADT) on a group of men who subsequently underwent radical prostatectomy. It is apparent from these data that those men who underwent ADT suffered worse sexual function outcomes. Unfortunately, preoperative International Index of Erectile Function data were not available, which represents a significant limitation of the course data. Furthermore, men treated with ADT were more likely to undergo non–nerve-sparing surgery; despite this, within-group comparisons indicate that within each group (bilateral, unilateral, and non–nerve-sparing surgery), men exposed to ADT fared worse.

The indications for neoadjuvant ADT should be carefully considered; whereas these data are by no means definitive, it cannot be safely assumed that even a short course of androgen deprivation is free of short- and long-term risks; therefore, this is not a treatment to be dispensed casually with the intent of "doing something while waiting for definitive therapy."

A. W. Shindel, MD

Intermittent versus Continuous Androgen Deprivation in Prostate Cancer
Hussain M, Tangen CM, Berry DL, et al (Univ of Michigan, Ann Arbor; Southwest Oncology Group Statistical Ctr, Seattle, WA; Dana-Farber Cancer Inst, Boston, MA; et al)
N Engl J Med 368:1314-1325, 2013

Background.—Castration resistance occurs in most patients with metastatic hormone-sensitive prostate cancer who are receiving androgen-deprivation therapy. Replacing androgens before progression of the disease is hypothesized to prolong androgen dependence.

Methods.—Men with newly diagnosed, metastatic, hormone-sensitive prostate cancer, a performance status of 0 to 2, and a prostate-specific antigen (PSA) level of 5 ng per milliliter or higher received a luteinizing hormone–releasing hormone analogue and an antiandrogen agent for 7 months. We then randomly assigned patients in whom the PSA level fell to 4 ng per milliliter or lower to continuous or intermittent androgen deprivation, with patients stratified according to prior or no prior hormonal

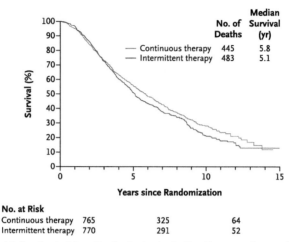

FIGURE 1.—Median Survival from Randomization in the Two Treatment Groups. (Reprinted from Hussain M, Tangen CM, Berry DL, et al. Intermittent versus continuous androgen deprivation in prostate cancer. *N Engl J Med.* 2013;368:1314-1325, Copyright 2013, with permission from Massachusetts Medical Society.)

therapy, performance status, and extent of disease (minimal or extensive). The coprimary objectives were to assess whether intermittent therapy was noninferior to continuous therapy with respect to survival, with a one-sided test with an upper boundary of the hazard ratio of 1.20, and whether quality of life differed between the groups 3 months after randomization.

Results.—A total of 3040 patients were enrolled, of whom 1535 were included in the analysis: 765 randomly assigned to continuous androgen deprivation and 770 assigned to intermittent androgen deprivation. The median follow-up period was 9.8 years. Median survival was 5.8 years in the continuous-therapy group and 5.1 years in the inter-mittent-therapy group (hazard ratio for death with intermittent therapy, 1.10; 90% confidence interval, 0.99 to 1.23). Intermittent therapy was associated with better erectile function and mental health ($P < 0.001$ and $P = 0.003$, respectively) at month 3 but not thereafter. There were no significant differences between the groups in the number of treatment-related high-grade adverse events.

Conclusions.—Our findings were statistically inconclusive. In patients with metastatic hormonesensitive prostate cancer, the confidence interval for survival exceeded the upper boundary for noninferiority, suggesting that we cannot rule out a 20% greater risk of death with intermittent therapy than with continuous therapy, but too few events occurred to rule out significant inferiority of intermittent therapy. Intermittent therapy resulted in small improvements in quality of life. (Funded by the National Cancer Institute and others; ClinicalTrials.gov number, NCT00002651.) (Fig 1).

▶ This important trial addresses an important issue for the care of men with metastatic prostate cancer—whether intermittent or continuous hormonal ablation is superior in terms of overall survival and quality of life. This trial was conducted as a noninferiority trial, and technically the results would say that intermittent hormonal therapy is not inferior to continuous therapy in terms of survival (Fig 1). But, because the relatively wide confidence interval of the hazard rate for mortality exceeded 1.2 (it was up to 1.23), there is a chance that intermittent therapy may be significantly (ie, more than 20%) worse. Intermittent therapy showed improved quality of life in terms of mental well-being and erectile function.

Given this study and the results of the Canadian Trial of intermittent vs continuous therapy in men with biochemical recurrence after primary therapy,[1] it seems that intermittent therapy is most appropriate for men with lower disease burden rather than "all comers" with metastatic disease. How this issue will be affected by use of currently available secondary and tertiary hormonal therapies (eg, enzalutamide and abiraterone) is unknown.

G. L. Andriole, Jr, MD

Reference

1. Crook JM, O'Callaghan CJ, Duncan G, et al. Intermittent androgen suppression for rising PSA level after radiotherapy. *N Engl J Med.* 2012;367:895-903.

Basic Science

Association Between Germline *HOXB13* G84E Mutation and Risk of Prostate Cancer

Akbari MR, Trachtenberg J, Lee J, et al (Women's College Hosp, Toronto, Ontario, Canada; Princess Margaret Hosp, Toronto, Ontario, Canada; Univ of Toronto, Ontario, Canada)
J Natl Cancer Inst 104:1260-1202, 2012

Recently, a G84E mutation in *HOXB13*, a gene involved in prostate development, was shown to be strongly associated with an increased risk of prostate cancer. To confirm this association in a screening setting, we conducted a case—control study and sequenced germline DNA from peripheral leukocytes of 1843 men diagnosed with prostate cancer (case subjects) and 2225 men without prostate cancer (control subjects) for mutations in *HOXB13*. Subjects (aged 40—94 years) were prescreened and underwent a prostate biopsy at two tertiary care centers in Canada. The frequency of *HOXB13* variants was determined in case subjects and control subjects by race, and odds ratios and 95% confidence intervals were based on 2 × 2 table analysis. All statistical tests were two-sided. Twelve men of white race were identified to be carriers of the G84E mutation. The G84E mutation was more frequent among white case subjects than among white control subjects (10 of 1525 [0.7%] vs 2 of 1757 [0.1%], $P = .01$) and was associated with an increased risk of prostate cancer (unadjusted odds ratio = 5.8, 95% confidence interval = 1.3 to 26.5, $P = .01$).

▶ We have been searching for the genetic cause of prostate cancer for almost 20 years. In this context, the discovery of the G84E mutation in *HOXB13* is an important discovery because it is one of the first familial prostate cancer genes.[1] The fact that patients with this risk allele were over 20 times more likely to have prostate cancer is a striking result. The question now is whether this will be useful in routine clinical practice. The answer is an unequivocal maybe. This article confirmed that germline variants in *HOXB13* are more common in men with prostate cancer than in men without it. However, this genetic marker is unlikely to be useful as a risk assessment tool. The primary problem is that the variant is not very common in either cases or controls. This means that it is noninformative in the majority of cases. To put it another way, it is worth testing all men in which 10 of roughly 1600 men will be positive—that is less than 1%. Only if it is used in combination with other variants will it be useful. A secondary problem is that it is not one variant, but several within the gene that may contribute to disease risk. Although this is a very important scientific finding, it does imply that to maximize clinical utility, we will have to sequence this gene in everyone undergoing a biopsy to identify all patients at increased risk. This is clearly a costly endeavor in 2012. However, to be blunt, in my opinion, this is the future. Risk assessment must be tied to genetics. However, there are still technical, epidemiologic, and yes, societal issues before this can become a part of routine clinical care.

A. S. Kibel, MD

Reference

1. Ewing CM, Ray AM, Lange EM, et al. Germline mutations in HOXB13 and prostate-cancer risk. N Engl J Med. 2012;366:141-149.

Chemoprevention/Neoadjuvant Therapy

The REDUCE Follow-Up Study: Low Rate of New Prostate Cancer Diagnoses Observed During a 2-Year, Observational, Followup Study of Men Who Participated in the REDUCE Trial
Grubb RL, Andriole GL, Somerville MC, et al (Washington Univ School of Medicine in St Louis, MO; GlaxoSmithKline, Research Triangle Park, NC; et al)
J Urol 189:871-877, 2013

Purpose.—The primary objective of the REDUCE (REduction by DUtasteride of prostate Cancer Events) Follow-Up Study was to collect data on the occurrence of newly diagnosed prostate cancers for 2 years beyond the 4-year REDUCE study.

Materials and Methods.—The 4-year REDUCE study evaluated prostate cancer risk reduction in men taking dutasteride. This 2-year observational study followed men from REDUCE with a clinic visit shortly after study conclusion and with up to 2 annual telephone calls during which patient reported data were collected regarding prostate cancer events, chronic medication use, prostate specific antigen levels and serious adverse events. No study drug was provided and all biopsies during the 2-year followup were performed for cause. The primary objective was to collect data on the occurrence of new biopsy detectable prostate cancers. Secondary end points included assessment of Gleason score and serious adverse events.

Results.—A total of 2,751 men enrolled in the followup study with numbers similar to those of the REDUCE former treatment groups (placebo and dutasteride). Few new prostate cancers were detected during the 2-year followup period in either former treatment group. A greater number of cancers were detected in the former dutasteride group than in the former placebo group (14 vs 7 cases). No Gleason score 8—10 prostate cancers were detected in either former treatment group based on central pathology review. No new safety issues were identified during the study.

Conclusions.—Two years of followup of the REDUCE study cohort demonstrated a low rate of new prostate cancer diagnoses in the former placebo and dutasteride treated groups. No new Gleason 8—10 cancers were detected.

▶ This report presents further follow-up of the (Reduction by Dutasteride of Prostate Cancer Events) REDUCE trial, which evaluated the use of dutasteride to reduce the detection of prostate cancer in men with baseline elevated prostate-specific antigen (PSA). During the course of the trial, there was a numeric increase in the number of Gleason 8—10 cancers in the dutasteride-treated men that was attributed to biases, including study design and prostate size at time of biopsy. This study shows that with further follow-up, there is no additional excess Gleason 8—10 disease, which one might have expected if dutasteride was actively promoting the development of these tumors. These data provide some reassurance that the high-grade issues associated with 5α-reductase inhibitors are likely related to biases rather than to promotion of aggressive cancer.

G. L. Andriole, Jr, MD

Dutasteride in localised prostate cancer management: the REDEEM randomised, double-blind, placebo-controlled trial

Fleshner NE, Lucia MS, Egerdie B, et al (Univ of Toronto, Ontario, Canada; Univ of Colorado School of Medicine, Aurora; Urology Associates/Urologic Med Res, Kitchener, Ontario, Canada; et al)
Lancet 379:1103-1111, 2012

Background.—We aimed to investigate the safety and efficacy of dutasteride, a 5α-reductase inhibitor, on prostate cancer progression in men with low-risk disease who chose to be followed up with active surveillance.

Methods.—In our 3 year, randomised, double-blind, placebo-controlled study, undertaken at 65 academic medical centres or outpatient clinics in North America, we enrolled men aged 48—82 years who had low-volume,

Gleason score 5—6 prostate cancer and had chosen to be followed up with active surveillance. We randomly allocated participants in a one-to-one ratio, stratified by site and in block sizes of four, to receive once-daily dutasteride 0·5 mg or matching placebo. Participants were followed up for 3 years, with 12-core prostate biopsy samples obtained after 18 months and 3 years. The primary endpoint was time to prostate cancer progression, defined as the number of days between the start of study treatment and the earlier of either pathological progression (in patients with ≥ 1 biopsy assessment after baseline) or therapeutic progression (start of medical therapy). This trial is registered with ClinicalTrials.gov, number NCT00363311.

Findings.—Between Aug 10, 2006, and March 26, 2007, we randomly allocated 302 participants, of whom 289 (96%) had at least one biopsy procedure after baseline and were included in the primary analysis. By 3 years, 54 (38%) of 144 men in the dutasteride group and 70 (48%) of 145 controls had prostate cancer progression (pathological or therapeutic; hazard ratio 0·62, 95% CI 0·43—0·89; $p = 0·009$). Incidence of adverse events was much the same between treatment groups. 35 (24%) men in the dutasteride group and 23 (15%) controls had sexual adverse events or breast enlargement or tenderness. Eight (5%) men in the dutasteride group and seven (5%) controls had cardiovascular adverse events, but there were no prostate cancer-related deaths or instances of metastatic disease.

Interpretation.—Dutasteride could provide a beneficial adjunct to active surveillance for men with low-risk prostate cancer.

▶ The concept behind active surveillance is that men with low-risk prostate cancer can be safely followed. Only the men whose disease progresses are in need of treatment. There are 2 progression events: those with pathological progression and those who cannot tolerate being on active surveillance. The REDEEM trial demonstrated that dutasteride decreases both events; fewer patients had pathologic progression and fewer patients decided to undergo treatment irrespective of the rebiopsy findings. Lastly, in addition, fewer patients actually had cancer on a repeat biopsy. To put it another way, dutasteride prevented the cancer from becoming more aggressive, it reassured patients they were doing the right thing, and it eradicated some low-volume disease. So why are we not prescribing dutasteride for all our active surveillance patients? Good question. The issues with the trial are both internal and external. First and foremost, this was an older population of patients with patients up to 81 years of age being enrolled, more of a watchful waiting than active surveillance cohort. A second issue is that the PCPT and REDUCE trials demonstrated a small increase in grade progression with the use of 5α-reductase inhibitors for prophylaxis. This resulted in a black box warning that has scared away many physicians from its use. Lastly, while the side effects are in general mild, in a patient population with essentially no symptoms, any side effects seem bothersome. I have to admit I rarely prescribe dutasteride in this setting. That is primarily driven by the increased side effects; however, in an active surveillance patient with a strong family history, this might be a good option.

A. S. Kibel, MD

Aspirin Use and the Risk of Prostate Cancer Mortality in Men Treated With Prostatectomy or Radiotherapy

Choe KS, Cowan JE, Chan JM, et al (Univ of Texas Southwestern Med Ctr, Dallas; Univ of California, San Francisco; et al)

J Clin Oncol 30:3540-3544, 2012

Purpose.—Experimental evidence suggests that anticoagulants (ACs) may inhibit cancer growth and metastasis, but clinical data have been limited. We investigated whether use of ACs was associated with the risk of death from prostate cancer.

Patients and Methods.—This study comprised 5,955 men in the Cancer of the Prostate Strategic Urologic Research Endeavor database with localized adenocarcinoma of the prostate treated with radical prostatectomy (RP) or radiotherapy (RT). Of them, 2,175 (37%) were receiving ACs (warfarin, clopidogrel, enoxaparin, and/or aspirin). The risk of prostate cancer—specific mortality (PCSM) was compared between the AC and non-AC groups.

Results.—After a median follow-up of 70 months, risk of PCSM was significantly lower in the AC group compared with the non-AC group (3% v 8% at 10 years; $P < .01$). The risks of disease recurrence and bone metastasis were also significantly lower. In a subgroup analysis by clinical risk category, the reduction in PCSM was most prominent in patients with high-risk disease (4% v 19% at 10 years; $P < .01$). The benefit from AC was present across treatment modalities (RT or RP). Analysis by type of AC medication suggested that the PCSM reduction was primarily associated with aspirin. Multivariable analysis indicated that aspirin use was independently associated with a lower risk of PCSM (adjusted hazard ratio, 0.43; 95% CI, 0.21 to 0.87; $P = .02$).

Conclusion.—AC therapy, particularly aspirin, was associated with a reduced risk of PCSM in men treated with RT or RP for prostate cancer. The association was most prominent in patients with high-risk disease.

▶ This well-done article demonstrates an association between anticoagulation use (aspirin [ASA], clopidogrel, warfarin) and decreased prostate cancer mortality following radical prostatectomy and radiation therapy. Ten-year mortality was 5% less for prostate cancer patients who were given anticoagulants. The benefit appeared to be greatest for ASA and, importantly, patients with high-risk disease benefited more than patients who had intermediate-risk disease, which in turn had more benefit than for those with low-risk disease. The clear benefit with disease risk demonstrates the patients at greatest risk benefit the most.

The most obvious and tempting conclusion is that ASA should be given to all our patients. Not so fast. There are some potential confounders in this article, only some of which are addressed by the authors. The most concerning is that patients on anticoagulation therapy could be more likely to die of other causes, because they clearly have other significant medical problems. Although the authors did do cumulative incidence analysis to control for this, what they could not control was the bias of the cause of death. The data on death were drawn primarily from death certificates. There is already a tendency for cause of death to be listed as cardiopulmonary in patients who died of other causes. My guess is that this false ascertainment of the cause of death might be higher in a cohort of patients with significant cardiac disease. It would be interesting to know if overall mortality was lower in anticoagulation patients.

I do think this study provides further evidence that ASA and other anticoagulants have the potential to decrease mortality from this disease. Because many men should be taking ASA for other causes, this just adds to the potential long-term benefits.

A. S. Kibel, MD

Laparoscopic Radical Prostatectomy

Mapping of Pelvic Lymph Node Metastases in Prostate Cancer
Joniau S, Van den Bergh L, Lerut E, et al (Univ Hosps Leuven, Belgium)
Eur Urol 63:450-458, 2013

Background.—Opinions about the optimal lymph node dissection (LND) template in prostate cancer differ. Drainage and dissemination patterns are not necessarily identical.

Objective.—To present a precise overview of the lymphatic drainage pattern and to correlate those findings with dissemination patterns. We also investigated the relationship between the number of positive lymph nodes (LN+) and resected lymph nodes (LNs) per region.

Design, setting, and participants.—Seventy-four patients with localized prostate adenocarcinoma were prospectively enrolled. Patients did not show suspect LNs on computed tomography scan and had an LN involvement risk of ≥10% but ≤35% (Partin tables) or a cT3 tumor.

Intervention.—After intraprostatic technetium-99m nanocolloid injection, patients underwent planar scintigraphy and single-photon emission computed tomography imaging. Then surgery was performed, starting with a sentinel node (SN) procedure and a superextended lymphadenectomy followed by radical prostatectomy.

Outcome Measurements and Statistical Analysis.—Distribution of scintigraphically detected SNs and removed SNs per region were registered. The number of LN+, as well as the percentage LN+ of the total number of removed LNs per region, was demonstrated in combining data of all patients. The impact of the extent of LND on N-staging and on the number of LN+ removed was calculated.

TABLE 2.—The Impact of the Extent of Lymph Node Dissection on Nodal Staging, Including a Proposed New Standard Extended Lymph Node Dissection Template Based on these Results

	N+ Patients Correctly Staged, no. (%, 95% CI)	N+ Patients in Whom All N+ Removed, no. (%, 95% CI)	N+ Removed, no. (%)	Nodes Removed, no., Median (IQR)
Obturator LND	16/34 (47, 29−62)	5/34 (15, 3−26)	23/91 (25)	6 (4−9)
Limited LND (external iliac plus obturator regions)	26/34 (76, 62−88)	10/34 (29, 15−44)	47/91 (52)	12 (8−17)
Extended LND (external and internal iliac plus obturator regions)	32/34 (94, 85−100)	26/34 (76, 62−88)	79/91 (87)	16 (10−21)
New suggested LND template (eLND plus presacral regions)	33/34 (97, 91−100)	30/34 (88, 76−97)	87/91 (96)	18 (12−23)
Superextended LND (eLND plus presacral plus common iliac regions)	33/34 (97, 91−100)	33/34 (97, 91−100)	90/91 (99)	21 (16−27)
Superextended LND plus SN	34/34 (100)	34/34 (100)	91/91 (100)	21 (16−27)

N+ = node-positive; CI = confidence interval; IQR = interquartile range; LND = lymph node dissection; eLND = extended lymph node dissection; SN = sentinel node.

Results and Limitations.—A total of 470 SNs were scintigraphically detected (median: 6; interquartile range [IQR]: 3−9), of which 371 SNs were removed (median: 4; IQR: 2.25−6). In total, 91 LN+ (median: 2; IQR: 1−3) were found in 34 of 74 patients. The predominant site for LN+ was the internal iliac region. An extended LND (eLND) would have correctly staged 32 of 34 patients but would have adequately removed all LN+ in only 26 of 34 patients. When adding the presacral region, these numbers increased to 33 of 34 and 30 of 34 patients, respectively.

Conclusions.—Standard eLND would have correctly staged the majority of LN + patients, but 13% of the LN + would have been missed. Adding the presacral LNs to the template should be considered to obtain a minimal template with maximal gain.

Note.—This manuscript was invited based on the 2011 European Association of Urology meeting in Vienna (Table 2).

▶ This important study provides guidance for the most appropriate extent of pelvic lymph node dissection in patients with prostate cancer and 10% or greater chance of nodal metastases. The standard obturator dissection would miss many men with metastases elsewhere. As shown in Table 2, extended dissections, including the presacral nodes, are necessary to detect all such men with metastases. This extended dissection can be accomplished with acceptable morbidity.

G. L. Andriole, Jr, MD

17 Bladder Cancer

Impact of a Bladder Cancer Diagnosis on Smoking Behavior
Bassett JC, Gore JL, Chi AC, et al (Univ of California, Los Angeles; Univ of Washington School of Medicine, Seattle)
J Clin Oncol 30:1871-1878, 2012

Purpose.—Bladder cancer is the second most common tobacco-related malignancy. A new bladder cancer diagnosis may be an opportunity to imprint smoking cessation. Little is known about the impact of a diagnosis of bladder cancer on patterns of tobacco use and smoking cessation among patients with incident bladder cancer.

Patients and Methods.—A simple random sample of noninvasive bladder cancer survivors diagnosed in 2006 was obtained from the California Cancer Registry. Respondents completed a survey on history of tobacco use, beliefs regarding bladder cancer risk factors, and physician influence on tobacco cessation. Respondents were compared by smoking status. Those respondents smoking at diagnosis were compared with general population controls obtained from the California Tobacco Survey to determine the impact of a diagnosis of bladder cancer on patterns of tobacco use.

Results.—The response rate was 70% (344 of 492 eligible participants). Most respondents (74%) had a history of cigarette use. Seventeen percent of all respondents were smoking at diagnosis. Smokers with a new diagnosis of bladder cancer were almost five times as likely to quit smoking as smokers in the general population (48% *v* 10%, respectively; *P* < .001). The bladder cancer diagnosis and the advice of the urologist were the reasons cited most often for cessation. Respondents were more likely to endorse smoking as a risk factor for bladder cancer when the urologist was the source of their understanding.

Conclusion.—The diagnosis of bladder cancer is an opportunity for smoking cessation. Urologists can play an integral role in affecting the patterns of tobacco use of those newly diagnosed.

▶ The striking thing about this article is that the patients with newly diagnosed bladder cancer were almost 5 times as likely to quit smoking as smokers in the general population (48% vs 10%, respectively; *P* < .001). The primary reason was the urologist encouraging them to quit. This demonstrates that the teachable moment is just that—an opportunity to teach and the patient to learn. Many urologists are nihilistic—"the patient knows he/she should stop." Others just don't think it their job to convince a patient. I personally believe that even if a minority quit right away, eventually with enough reinforcement, patients will quit. This article provides evidence that, like water wearing away at a rock, every drop counts! I encourage everyone reading this to at least mention smoking cessation to his or her bladder cancer patient. Don't get preachy; just tell the facts. Don't just focus on bladder cancer. Mention heart disease, lung cancer, and—yes—impotence. You will be amazed at how many patients decide to quit. Maybe not right away, but eventually.

A. S. Kibel, MD

Routine Urine Cytology has No Role in Hematuria Investigations

Mishriki SF, Aboumarzouk O, Vint R, et al (Aberdeen Royal Infirmary Hosp, Scotland; et al)

J Urol 189:1255-1259, 2013

Purpose.—Urine cytology has been a long-standing first line investigation for hematuria and is recommended in current major guidelines. We determined the contribution of urine cytology in hematuria investigations and its cost implications.

Materials and Methods.—Data were prospectively collected for 2,778 consecutive patients investigated for hematuria at a United Kingdom teaching hospital from January 1999 to September 2007 with final analysis in October 2010. All patients underwent standard hematuria investigations including urine cytology, flexible cystoscopy and renal tract ultrasound with excretory urogram or computerized tomography urogram performed in those with visible hematuria without a diagnosis after first line tests. Patients with positive urine cytology as the only finding underwent further cystoscopy, retrograde studies or ureteroscopy with biopsy under general anesthesia. Outcomes in terms of eventual diagnosis were cross-referenced with initial urine cytology results (classified as malignant, suspicious, atypical, benign or unsatisfactory). Costs of urine cytology were calculated.

Results.—Of the patients 124 (4.5%) had malignant cells and 260 (9.4%) had atypical/suspicious results. For urothelial cancer cytology demonstrated 45.5% sensitivity and 89.5% specificity. Two patients with urine cytology as the only positive finding had urothelial malignancy on further investigation. For the entire cohort the cost of cytology was £111,120.

Conclusions.—Routine urine cytology is costly and of limited clinical value as a first line investigation for all patients with hematuria, and should be omitted from guidelines.

▶ Standard hematuria investigation includes imaging of the upper tract parenchyma and the urinary collecting system and cystourethroscopy. The utility of urinary cytology is dependent on the timing and method of urine collection as well as the experience of the cytopathologist. The specificity of a positive sample is very high, but the sensitivity is highly variable and is related to tumor grade. The low sensitivity should decrease its use in screening in all but those with a high risk for transitional cell cancer. Routine cytology is ill-advised because it adds little to the standard evaluation. In this prospective study, only 2 of 2778 patients had a negative cystoscopy, normal upper tract imaging, and a positive cytology with subsequent identification of transitional cell carcinoma. The false-positives result in unnecessary investigations. Although not evaluated in this study, other biomarkers, such as NMP 22, ImmunoCyt, and FISH increase sensitivity but sacrifice specificity and are best utilized in the follow-up of patients with known transitional cell cancer.

D. E. Coplen, MD

18 Urinary Reconstruction

Bladder Neck Closure in Conjunction with Enterocystoplasty and Mitrofanoff Diversion for Complex Incontinence: Closing the Door for Good
Kavanagh A, Afshar K, Scott H, et al (Univ of British Columbia, Vancouver, Canada)
J Urol 188:1561-1565, 2012

Purpose.—Bladder neck closure is an irreversible procedure requiring compliance with catheterization of a cutaneous stoma and historically has been reserved for the definitive treatment of intractable incontinence after prior failed procedures. We assessed long-term outcomes of our patients undergoing bladder neck closure including continence status, additional surgical interventions, postoperative complications, conception and sexual function, and satisfaction with bladder neck closure.

Materials and Methods.—We performed a retrospective review of all patients who underwent bladder neck closure between 1990 and 2010 at our institution.

Results.—A total of 28 consecutive patients (exstrophy 15 and neurogenic bladder 13 [myelomeningocele 4, cloacal anomaly 4, spinal cord injury 2, VACTERL (Vertebral Anorectal Cardiac Tracheo-Esophageal Radial Renal Limb) 1, sacral agenesis 1 and urogenital sinus 1]) were identified. Of these patients 19 (68%) had undergone 20 unsuccessful bladder neck procedures before bladder neck closure. Bladder neck closure was initially successful in 27 of the 28 (96.4%) patients. One patient required subsequent closure of a postoperative vesicovaginal fistula. Median time from bladder neck closure was 69 months (range 16 to 250). In 11 patients 16 additional procedures were required, including stomal injection of bulking agents (2), stomal revision for stenosis (2) or prolapse (1), percutaneous nephrolithotripsy for stone (1), open cystolithotomy (2), extracorporeal shock wave lithotripsy for upper tract stones (4), repair of augment rupture (3) and open retrograde ureteral stenting for stone (1). The total surgical reintervention rate was 39.3% (11 of 28). There were no observed cases of progressive or de novo hydronephrosis.

Conclusions.—Bladder neck closure in conjunction with enterocystoplasty and Mitrofanoff diversion is an effective means of achieving continence in complex cases as a primary or secondary therapy. Long-term urological followup into adulthood is essential.

▶ This small case series illustrates a number of points. First, these are a complex group of patients. Second, achieving continence comes at the cost of several subsequent procedures to address other genitourinary issues as they arise. Third, and most important, these patients require long-term follow-up. It could be argued that these patients are only at the beginning of their need for long-term follow-up. This cohort of patients represents a group of children initially treated for their incontinence (82% of whom underwent bladder neck closure and diversion as an adult). Thus their life expectancy and potential for other complications and interventions in the future is quite expansive.

E. S. Rovner, MD

Half Century of Followup After Ureterosigmoidostomy Performed in Early Childhood

Pettersson L, Tranberg J, Abrahamsson K, et al (Hallands Hosp Halmstad, Sweden; Queen Silvia Children's Hosp, Gothenburg, Sweden; et al)
J Urol 189:1870-1875, 2013

Purpose.—We studied clinical outcomes, especially regarding colorectal adenocarcinoma, in patients who underwent ureterosigmoidostomy in early childhood between 1944 and 1961.

Materials and Methods.—A total of 25 consecutive patients underwent ureterosigmoidostomy at a mean age of 3.1 years. The most common indication for ureterosigmoidostomy was bladder exstrophy-epispadias complex. The study period ended in 2010. Patient files were retrospectively evaluated, personal telephone interviews were performed and colorectal histology was reevaluated. One girl who died 4 days postoperatively was excluded.

Results.—Of the 24 patients 17 were alive in 2010 with a mean age of 59 years (range 48 to 67), and 2 still had a functioning ureterosigmoidostomy. A total of 20 patients with a mean age of 33 years had undergone re-diversion at a mean of 30 years postoperatively. Invasive colorectal adenocarcinoma developed in 7 patients and colorectal adenocarcinoma in situ in 1. Five patients died due to generalized colorectal adenocarcinoma. Mean time from ureterosigmoidostomy to diagnosis of invasive colorectal adenocarcinoma was 38 years (range 23 to 55). Three cases were diagnosed at 1, 21 and 25 years after re-diversion. One patient with colorectal adenocarcinoma in situ was 22 years old at polyp resection, which was 20 years after re-diversion. A carcinoid tumor developed in 1 patient. Of the 7 cases of invasive colorectal adenocarcinoma 6 were low differentiated.

Conclusions.—After a half century of followup in 25 individuals undergoing ureterosigmoidostomy during childhood 17 were still alive and 20 had undergone re-diversion. Compared to the general Swedish population, the risk of colorectal adenocarcinoma was increased 42 times and the incidence of low differentiation was extremely high.

▶ The authors report very long-term follow-up after ureterosigmoidostomy that was performed in infancy (mean, 3.1 years). In all but 4 children, the diversion was performed in infants with exstrophy/epispadias complex. The risk of colorectal adenocarcinoma in these patients was 42 times higher after ureterosigmoidostomy than in the general Swedish population. Cancer did not develop in any patient before 20 years after diversion. Given this time lag, ureterosigmoidostomy may be used as a temporary diversion for 15 to 20 years without increasing the risk of colorectal cancer. Unfortunately, routine colonoscopy did not detect 2 tumors because the growth was in the ureter. Upper tract imaging with a computed tomography scan or magnetic resonance urogram is required in addition to endoscopic evaluation. Two of the patients who died from colorectal cancer had recurrence at the ureteroenteric anastomotic site that was not resected at the time of rediversion. Radical resection of this site is required when a ureterosigmoidostomy is taken down. Ureterosigmoidostomy may be an option in adult patients with a life expectancy of less than 20 years. This article should be reviewed by urologists performing reconstruction and taking care of exstrophy/epispadias patients.

D. E. Coplen, MD

19 Infertility

Sperm counts and endocrinological markers of spermatogenesis in long-term survivors of testicular cancer
Brydøy M, for the Norwegian Urology Cancer Group (NUCG) III study group
(Univ of Bergen, Norway; et al)
Br J Cancer 107:1833-1839, 2012

Background.—The objective of this study was to assess markers of spermatogenesis in long-term survivors of testicular cancer (TC) according to treatment, and to explore correlations between the markers and associations with achieved paternity following TC treatment.

Methods.—In 1191 TC survivors diagnosed between 1980 and 1994, serum-follicle stimulating hormone (s-FSH; $n = 1191$), s-inhibin B ($n = 441$), and sperm counts (millions per ml; $n = 342$) were analysed in a national follow-up study in 1998-2002. Paternity was assessed by a questionnaire.

Results.—At median 11 years follow-up, 44% had oligo- (<15 millions per ml; 29%) or azoospermia (15%). Sperm counts and s-inhibin B were significantly lower and s-FSH was higher after chemotherapy, but not after radiotherapy (RT), when compared with surgery only. All measures were significantly more abnormal following high doses of chemotherapy (cisplatin (Cis) >850 mg, absolute cumulative dose) compared with lower doses (Cis ≤850 mg). Sperm counts were moderately correlated with s-FSH (−0.500), s-inhibin B (0.455), and s-inhibin B: FSH ratio (−0.524; all $P < 0.001$). All markers differed significantly between those who had achieved post-treatment fatherhood and those with unsuccessful attempts.

Conclusion.—The RT had no long-term effects on the assessed markers of spermatogenesis, whereas chemotherapy had. At present, the routine evaluation of s-inhibin B adds little in the initial fertility evaluation of TC survivors.

▶ This article evaluates spermatogenesis in a known subfertile population. Paternity was determined by questionnaire, and those utilizing pretreatment cryopreserved semen were excluded from the analysis. Radiation therapy has no apparent long-term effect on spermatogenesis. Chemotherapy clearly has a long-term effect that is dose related. Although surgery (retroperitoneal lymph node dissection) alone does not affect spermatogenesis, it may adversely impact ejaculation and alter fertility potential. Table 3 in the original article shows the clear relationship between serum follicle-stimulating hormone, sperm counts, and paternity. The paternity rate was reduced 50% in those receiving high-dose cisplatin when compared with the surgery-alone and radiation groups. It is very encouraging that despite the history of testicular cancer, 66% of men attempting paternity were successful without using cryopreserved sperm.

D. E. Coplen, MD

Predictors of Spermatogenesis in Orchiectomy Specimens

Choy JT, Wiser HJ, Bell SW, et al (Northwestern Univ Feinberg School of Medicine, Chicago, IL; Southern Illinois Univ School of Medicine, Springfield; Saint John's Hosp, Springfield, IL)
Urology 81:288-292, 2013

Objective.—To evaluate the presence of spermatogenesis in orchiectomy specimens of patients with testicular cancer to determine possible predictors of success with oncologic testicular sperm extraction of the cancerous testis at orchiectomy.

Materials and Methods.—We retrospectively reviewed the pathology reports and slides from 83 men who underwent radical orchiectomy for testicular cancer at 2 institutions from 1999 to 2010. The presence or absence of spermatogenesis in each specimen was determined. Data on tumor histopathologic type, serum tumor markers, and tumor size were also obtained and analyzed to detect any associations with the presence of spermatogenesis.

Results.—The 83 specimens included 41 pure seminomas, 36 nonseminomatous and mixed germ cell tumors, and 6 benign lesions. Overall, spermatogenesis was detected in 48 of 77 (62%) cancerous specimens. Spermatogenesis was present in 22 of 41 (54%) pure seminomas and 26 of 36 (72%) nonseminomatous and mixed germ cell tumors, with no significant difference found between the 2 subtypes ($P = .11$). No association was found between tumor marker levels and the presence of spermatogenesis. A logistic regression model revealed a statistically significant inverse relationship between tumor size and spermatogenesis presence ($P = .004$).

Conclusion.—At orchiectomy, most cancerous testes contained active spermatogenesis and, thus, represent a viable source for sperm cryopreservation with oncologic testicular sperm extraction. A small tumor size proved to be a positive prognostic indicator for the presence of spermatogenesis, although a larger tumor size did not preclude the presence of spermatogenesis.

▶ Patients with testicular cancer often are subfertile. The return of spermatogenesis after definitive and nearly always successful definitive therapy is unpredictable. Sperm banking and cryopreservation before initiation of treatment are advised. The authors propose the theoretical application of oncologic testicular sperm extraction in cases in which a pretreatment sperm sample is not readily retrieved. The authors retrospectively evaluated orchiectomy specimens, and spermatogenesis was identified in most men irrespective of histopathology, tumor marker levels, and tumor size. It is unclear if pretreatment gonadotropins (luteinizing hormone/follicle-stimulating hormone) and testosterone would better identify the subpopulation with retrievable sperm. This appears to be a viable option for fertility preservation given the current success of ICSI.

D. E. Coplen, MD

Seminal and molecular evidence that sauna exposure affects human spermatogenesis

Garolla A, Torino M, Sartini B, et al (Univ of Padova, Italy)
Hum Reprod 28:877-885, 2013

Study Question.—What are the effects of continuous sauna exposure on seminal parameters, sperm chromatin, sperm apoptosis and expression of genes involved in heat stress and hypoxia?

Summary Answer.—Scrotal hyperthermia by exposure to sauna can induce a significant alteration of spermatogenesis.

What is Known Already.—Several authors have evidenced that high temperature has dramatic effects on spermatogenesis.

Study Design, Size and Duration.—A longitudinal time-course study. Data from 10 subjects exposed to Finnish sauna were collected before sauna (T0), after 3 months of sauna sessions (T1) and after 3 (T2) and 6 months (T3) from the end of sauna exposure.

Participants/Materials, Setting and Methods.—Ten normozoospermic volunteers underwent two sauna sessions per week for 3 months, at 80–90°C, each lasting 15 min. Sex hormones, sperm parameters, sperm chromatin structure, sperm apoptosis and expression of genes involved in heat stress and hypoxia were evaluated at the start, at the end of sauna exposure and after 3 and 6 months from sauna discontinuation. Student's *t*-test for paired data was used for statistical analysis.

Main Results and the Role of Chance.—At the end of sauna exposure, we found a strong impairment of sperm count and motility ($P < 0.001$), while no significant change in sex hormones was present. Decreases in the percentage of sperm with normal histone-protamine substitution (78.7 ± 4.5 versus 69.0 ± 4.1), chromatin condensation (70.7 ± 4.7 versus 63.6 ± 3.3) and mitochondrial function (76.8 ± 4.9 versus 54.0 ± 6.1) were also evident at T1, and strong parallel up-regulation of genes involved in response to heat stress and hypoxia was found. All these effects were completely reversed at T3.

Limitations and Reasons for Caution.—Absence of subjects with abnormal sperm parameters was the major limitation of this study.

Wider Implications of the Findings.—Our data demonstrated for the first time that in normozoospermic subjects, sauna exposure induces a significant but reversible impairment of spermatogenesis, including alteration of sperm parameters, mitochondrial function and sperm DNA packaging. The large use of Finnish sauna in Nordic countries and its growing use in other parts of the world make it important to consider the impact of this lifestyle choice on men's fertility.

Study Funding/Competing Interest(s).—No external funding was sought for this study and the authors have no conflict of interest to declare.

▶ In most mammals, the testes reside outside the body because spermatogenesis is optimal at temperatures below the natural body temperature. There is increasing interest in the hypothesis that environmental, occupational, and lifestyle choices can impair testicular function. Fig 2 in the original article demonstrates changes in seminal parameters after sauna exposure. The changes were not associated with alteration of sex hormones (follicle-stimulating hormone, luteinizing hormone, testosterone, and inhibin), so it is unclear whether the perturbation correlates with decreased fertility. The upregulation of genes involved in heat stress and hypoxia may represent a stress response and a mechanism to preserve spermatogenesis.

D. E. Coplen, MD

Parental attitudes toward fertility preservation in boys with cancer: context of different risk levels of infertility and success rates of fertility restoration

Sadri-Ardekani H, Akhondi M-M, Vossough P, et al (Avicenna Res Inst, Tehran, Iran; Mahak Childhood Cancer Hosp, Tehran, Iran; et al)
Fertil Steril 99:796-802, 2013

Objective.—To measure the parental attitudes toward fertility preservation in boys with cancer.

Design.—Retrospective cohort study.

Setting.—Questionnaire survey via regular mail.

Patient(s).—A total of 465 families whose sons were already treated for cancer.

Intervention(s).—The questionnaire was designed for two groups based on child's age at the time of cancer diagnosis: <12 and ≥12 years old.

Main Outcome Measure(s).—Descriptive statistics regarding a positive or negative attitude of parents toward fertility preservation options in the context of different risk levels of infertility and success rates of fertility restoration.

Result(s).—The response rate was 78%. Sixty-four percent of parents of boys ≥12 years old would agree to store sperm obtained by masturbation and/or electroejaculation, and 54% of parents of boys <12 years old would agree to store a testicular biopsy. If the risk of infertility or the success rate of fertility restoration were ≤20%, more than one-fourth of parents would still opt for fertility preservation.

Conclusion(s).—All parents should be counseled about the risks of infertility due to cancer treatment, because many parents want to preserve their son's fertility even if the risk of becoming infertile or the chances on fertility restoration are low.

▶ Gonadal failure and poor long-term reproductive outcomes are adverse events related to treatment of childhood cancer. In postpubertal males, sperm retrieval and cryopreservation from ejaculate is the preferred option. Testicular biopsy and extraction is an option when cultural sensitivities preclude masturbation. Cryopreservation of testicular tissue (and spermatogonial stem cells) is required in prepubertal males. This is technically possible, although further work is required for subsequent transplantation or engraftment to be clinically available.

Only 22% of parents were aware of the relationship between cancer treatment and infertility, so parental counseling regarding this possibility is imperative. As expected, parental understanding was directly related to their level of education. Most parents would intervene regardless if the risk of infertility was small or the chance of preservation of fertility was small. A team approach is required to support boys with cancer and to facilitate informed decisions regarding fertility preservation.

D. E. Coplen, MD

Outcomes of the management of post-chemotherapy retroperitoneal lymph node dissection-associated anejaculation
Hsiao W, Deveci S, Mulhall JP (Memorial Sloan-Kettering Cancer Ctr, NY; Weill Cornell Med College, NY)
BJU Int 110:1196-1200, 2012

What's Known on the Subject? and What Does the Study Add?.—Modern surgical techniques have allowed preservation of fertility in most patients after post-chemotherapy retroperitoneal lymph node dissection (PC-RPLND), but some patients still have infertility after surgery. We reviewed our experience treating infertility in 26 men after PC-RPLND. Using a structured clinical pathway we obtained sperm in 81% of men for use in assisted reproduction.

Objective.—•To evaluate the effectiveness of a clinical pathway on sperm retrieval outcomes in patients presenting with infertility after post-chemotherapy (PC) retroperitoneal lymph node dissection (RPLND).

Patients and Methods.—•We carried out a retrospective review of patients with advanced testicular cancer, presenting with infertility after PC-RPLND in a large reproductive urology practice.

•We implemented a clinical pathway where pseudoephedrine was first administered. If this medication failed, electroejaculation (EEJ) and/or testicular sperm extraction (TESE) was carried out.

•The primary outcome was retrieval of sperm for use in assisted reproduction.

Results.—•Four men had retrograde ejaculation, of whom two converted to antegrade ejaculation with medical therapy.

•In all, 22 patients had failure of emission (FOE) and, of these, no patient converted to antegrade ejaculation with medication.

•In patients with FOE, sperm was found in 15/20 of those experiencing a successful EEJ.

•Seven patients underwent TESE for azoospermia on EEJ or no ejaculate on EEJ, three of whom had sperm found on TESE.

•Sperm was found for assisted reproduction in 81% (21/26) patients.

Conclusions.—•There appears to be no role for the use of pseudoephedrine therapy in patients with FOE after PC-RPLND.

•The use of a structured clinical pathway may optimize patient care.

▶ Nerve-sparing techniques have been developed to spare the hypogastric plexus during retroperitoneal lymph node dissection. However, postchemotherapy fibrosis makes nerve identification and preservation difficult. Anejaculation is an unfortunate complication related to disruption of sympathetic outflow. A small number of men have retrograde ejaculation, and sperm can be harvested from the bladder after ejaculation. An alpha agonist may close the bladder neck and facilitate antegrade flow. Most men have failure of emission that can be treated with electroejaculation (EEJ) or testicular sperm extraction (TESE).

Fig 3 in the original article shows the structured clinical pathway used in this study. It is unclear if a different alpha agonist like imipramine would have higher efficacy. The authors feel that EEJ is the preferred initial approach because it was successful in the majority and is less invasive than TESE. There is no outcome reported regarding the quality of the sperm and eventual fertilization.

D. E. Coplen, MD

Does Infertility Treatment Increase Male Reproductive Tract Disorder?

Bang JK, Lyu SW, Choi J, et al (CHA Univ, Seoul, Korea)
Urology 81:644-648, 2013

Objective.—To determine the association between assisted human reproduction and male reproductive disorders in infants conceived by this means.

Materials and Methods.—Between January 2008 and December 2011, 15,332 neonates were born in our hospital. We assessed the birth weight, gestational age, and other characteristics of the 7752 male infants and determined the association between methods of conception and male reproductive disorders in the infants. We also analyzed the influence of male factor on the occurrence of these disorders.

Results.—Ninety-nine newborns (1.3%) were diagnosed with cryptorchidism, 8 (0.1%) were diagnosed with hypospadias, and 4 (0.05%) were diagnosed with both. Cryptorchidism was more common in children conceived through in vitro fertilization (IVF) and IVF/intracytoplasmic sperm injection (IVF/ICSI; $P < .05$), and hypospadias was more common in children conceived through IVF/ICSI ($P < .05$). Children conceived through intrauterine insemination (IUI), IVF, and IVF/ICSI had higher rates of low birth weight and preterm birth. Logistic regression analysis showed that low birth weight and preterm birth were significantly associated with male reproductive disorders, whereas the method of conception was not. Male factor was not significantly associated with these disorders.

Conclusion.—IVF and IVF/ICSI increase the risks of low birth weight and preterm birth, resulting in increased rates of hypospadias and cryptorchidism. Male factor was not associated with reproductive disorders in male infants.

▶ Population-based studies show an increased incidence of hypospadias over the last 20 to 30 years. This may be related to environmental exposures (phytoestrogens and other chemicals that are endocrine disrupters). An association has also been shown with low birth weight, advanced maternal age, assisted reproductive techniques, and multiple gestation pregnancies. As shown in this study, there is a statistically higher incidence of all of these risk factors when assisted reproductive techniques are used.

Undescended testis and hypospadias were statistically more likely in the 15% of infants conceived after in vitro fertilization or intracytoplasmic sperm injection. However, regression analysis shows that preterm birth and low birth weight are actually the independent predictors. This is a large study of more than 15 000 births. The number of boys with cryptorchidism and hypospadias is very small because the overall incidence is low. This may impact the accuracy of the conclusions.

D. E. Coplen, MD

20 Varicocele

Pubertal Screening and Treatment for Varicocele do not Improve Chance of Paternity as Adult
Bogaert G, Orye C, De Win G (Univ Hosp Leuven, Belgium)
J Urol 189:2298-2304, 2013

Purpose.—We investigated the eventual positive effects of early screening and treatment for varicocele in pubertal boys without symptoms to determine their chance of paternity later in life. It has not been proved if the presence of varicocele during puberty has an influence on later fertility or paternity. However, since an influence is believed to exist, beginning in 1987 the Belgian Society of Pediatrics has recommended screening all boys 12 to 17 years old during their yearly medical examination and referral for followup or treatment if varicocele is detected. At our clinic patients and their parents were informed about and able to choose between varicocele treatment (antegrade sclerotherapy) and observation. We subsequently contacted these patients, who are now older than 30 years, and inquired about their paternity.

Materials and Methods.—We selected for this study pubertal boys 12 to 17 years old with a varicocele who were referred by screening pediatricians to our pediatric urology clinic between 1989 and 2005. We excluded patients with bilateral or unilateral right varicocele and patients with other medical problems that could influence fertility. A total of 661 patients were eligible for the study. Minimally invasive treatment of varicocele, ie antegrade sclerotherapy (with the patient under local or general anesthesia), was offered but not required. Of the patients 372 underwent treatment (mean age 15.3 years, median 15.6) and 289 were followed conservatively (mean age 17.1, median 16.4). All patients were contacted twice by letter and, if no response was received, once by telephone. Patients were asked about paternity, time to conception and whether they had visited a fertility center.

Results.—Of the 361 respondents 158 (43%) had an active desire to have a child. Paternity was achieved in 85% of the conservatively followed group and 78% of the active treatment group ($p > 0.05$).

Conclusions.—There is no beneficial effect of pubertal screening and treatment for varicocele regarding chance of paternity later in life.

▶ There is an increased prevalence of varicocele (20%–30% vs 10%–15% in the general population) in men presenting for infertility evaluation. The authors retrospectively report on a nonrandomized and poorly controlled comparison of observation vs antegrade sclerotherapy (repair performed via a small scrotal incision for the treatment of varicocele).

Because most adolescents with a varicocele are not attempting paternity, evaluation typically focuses on discrepant testicular size as an indication for intervention. Semen analysis is rarely obtained in adolescents and is not necessarily predictive of fertility potential. In this study, only 8% of treated patients had a smaller testicle at the time of intervention. It is unclear why the others were treated, but if size discrepancy is a surrogate for future fertility issues, then the study population becomes very small. A subset analysis of the 27 boys with size discrepancy shows no difference in paternity in the 2 groups (14 of 17 in the treated group and 9 of 10 in the observed group).

The excellent paternity in both sets confirms what we already know. Eight percent of men with a varicocele have normal fertility and can father a child. Because there is no serial data on testicular size and no seminal data, this study does not help us discern the 20% of adolescents with a varicocele who will have fertility issues. Because it is not known whether pre-emptive varicocelectomy is better than one performed after an infertility evaluation confirms an abnormal semen analysis, an observational approach to the adolescent varicocele is very reasonable.

D. E. Coplen, MD

21 Pediatric Urology

Finasteride for recurrent priapism in children and adolescents: A report on 5 cases
Barroso U Jr, Marques TC, Novaes HF (Escola Bahiana de Medicina e Saúde Pública, Brazil)
Int Braz J Urol 38:682-686, 2012

Purpose.—Recurrent priapism is prevalent in children. Different medications have been used to avoid new episodes, however, there is no consensus regarding the best option. The use of finasteride to treat priapism in adults has already been tested. The aim of the present study was to test the hypothesis that a low dose of finasteride would be effective in preventing recurrent priapism in children.

Materials and Methods.—Since 2007, five children and adolescents with recurrent episodes of priapism have been treated with finasteride in our department, and the medical records of these patients were reviewed for this study. In four cases, the dose used was 1 mg a day, while the remaining patient used 1 mg twice a day.

Results.—Prior to initiating finasteride treatment, one patient reported having had 6 episodes of acute priapism, while the remaining patients had more than 10 episodes. One of the patients reported having stuttering priapism almost daily. With a mean follow-up of 20 months, four patients had no episodes and only one patient complained of sporadic and shorter duration episodes.

Conclusions.—These initial results suggest that a low daily dose of finasteride appears to represent an effective and safe form of treatment for recurrent priapism in children and adolescents with SCD. However, in order to confirm these initial findings, studies with a large population and a control group are essential.

▶ Recurrent priapism in sickle cell disease can be a significant problem that results in multiple emergency room visits/hospitalizations for irrigation and aspiration when conservative measures (eg, hydration, oxygen, analgesics) fail. Corporal fibrosis and impotence are long-term effects of recurrent episodes. The American Urological Association guidelines support the use of androgen disruption (luteinizing hormone-releasing hormone [LHRH] analogs, androgen receptor blockers, and suppression of production) to prevent recurrent priapism in adults. This approach potentially decreases libido and sexual function.

The severity of the prior priapism episodes in the patient population in this study is not clear. The Tanner stage is not listed, but presumably at least 2 of the boys ages 8 and 10 were prepubertal. Because these boys have an undetectable testosterone level, it is unclear why blockage of 5-α reductase would decrease the frequency of priapism in these boys. It is also unclear why the incidence remained low after the medication was stopped. Finasteride may be less expensive and easier to administer than an LHRH analog, but compliance with daily administration in an adolescent population may be low. Further evaluation of the efficacy in a controlled setting is indicated.

D. E. Coplen, MD

22 Antenatal Hydronephrosis

Risk Factors for Renal Injury in Children With a Solitary Functioning Kidney
Westland R, Kurvers RA, van Wijk JAE, et al (VU Univ Med Ctr, Amsterdam, Netherlands; Radboud Univ Nijmegen Med Ctr, Netherlands)
Pediatrics 131:e478-e485, 2013

Objective.—The hyperfiltration hypothesis implies that children with a solitary functioning kidney are at risk to develop hypertension, proteinuria, and chronic kidney disease. We sought to determine the presenting age of renal injury and identify risk factors for children with a solitary functioning kidney.

Methods.—We evaluated 407 patients for signs of renal injury, defined as hypertension, proteinuria, an impaired glomerular filtration rate, and/or the use of renoprotective medication. Patients were subdivided on the basis of type of solitary functioning kidney and the presence of ipsilateral congenital anomalies of the kidney and urinary tract (CAKUT). The development of renal injury was analyzed with Kaplan-Meier analysis. Risk factors were identified by using logistic regression models.

Results.—Renal injury was found in 37% of all children. Development of renal injury increased by presence of ipsilateral CAKUT (odds ratio [OR] 1.66; $P = .04$) and age (OR 1.09; $P < .001$). Renal length was inversely associated with the risk to develop renal injury (OR 0.91; $P = .04$). In all patients, the median time to renal injury was 14.8 years (95% confidence interval 13.7–16.0 years). This was significantly shortened for patients with ipsilateral CAKUT (12.8 years, 95% confidence interval 10.6–15.1 years).

Conclusions.—Our study determines independent risk factors for renal injury in children with a solitary functioning kidney. Because many children develop renal injury, we emphasize the need for clinical follow-up in these patients starting at birth.

▶ Patients with an acquired solitary kidney are at high risk for renal injury when the contralateral kidney was removed for reflux, urinary obstruction, or other anomalies of the urinary tract. Presumably, this is related to similar pathology in the ipsilateral kidney. It is somewhat surprising that 31% of patients with a congenitally solitary kidney (renal agenesis or multicystic dysplastic kidney) had renal injury that was identifiable in childhood. This is likely related to the high incidence of ipsilateral anomalies (42%), reflux (20%), and urinary tract infections (48%) in the study group. Because the patient population was followed up at tertiary care medical centers, there may be a selection bias for children with more significant renal abnormalities. An infant with compensatory enlargement (> 95th percentile for length) and normal corticomedullary differentiation is at low risk for development of renal injury. In these cases, follow-up with blood pressure, urine dipstick for proteinuria, and a serum creatinine level in a couple of years is reasonable. Obviously, infants with identifiable ipsilateral abnormalities need closer follow-up.

D. E. Coplen, MD

Antibiotic Prophylaxis for Urinary Tract Infections in Antenatal Hydronephrosis

Braga LH, Mijovic H, Farrokhyar F, et al (McMaster Univ, Hamilton, Ontario, Canada; et al)
Pediatrics 131:e251-e261, 2013

Background and Objective.—Continuous antibiotic prophylaxis (CAP) is recommended to prevent urinary tract infections (UTIs) in newborns with antenatal hydronephrosis (HN). However, there is a paucity of high-level evidence supporting this practice. The goal of this study was to conduct a systematic evaluation to determine the value of CAP in reducing the rate of UTIs in this patient population.

Methods.—Pertinent articles and abstracts from 4 electronic databases and gray literature, spanning publication dates between 1990 and 2010, were included. Eligibility criteria included studies of children <2 years old with antenatal HN, receiving either CAP or not, and reporting on development of UTIs, capturing information on voiding cystourethrogram (VCUG) result and HN grade. Full-text screening and quality appraisal were conducted by 2 independent reviewers.

Results.—Of 1681 citations, 21 were included in the final analysis ($N = 3876$ infants). Of these, 76% were of moderate or low quality. Pooled UTI rates in patients with low-grade HN were similar regardless of CAP status: 2.2% on prophylaxis versus 2.8% not receiving prophylaxis. In children with high-grade HN, patients receiving CAP had a significantly lower UTI rate versus those not receiving CAP (14.6% [95% confidence interval: 9.3-22.0] vs 28.9% [95% confidence interval: 24.6−33.6], $P < 01$). The estimated number needed to treat to prevent 1 UTI in patients with high-grade HN was 7.

Conclusions.—This systematic review suggests value in offering CAP to infants with high-grade HN, however the impact of important variables (eg, gender, reflux, circumcision status) could not be assessed. The overall level of evidence of available data is unfortunately moderate to low.

▶ The value of antibiotic prophylaxis in infants with a history of urinary tract infection and vesicoureteral reflux is widely debated. Randomized trials in infants older than 6 months show some benefit in girls and in the presence of high-grade reflux. This meta-analysis evaluates the utility of prophylaxis in asymptomatic infants with prenatally identified renal dilation. Renal pelvic dilation and minimal caliectasis were classified as low-grade antenatal hydronephrosis (HN), whereas diffuse caliectasis with or without cortical thinning was classified as high-grade HN.

The forest plots in Figs 2 and 3 in the original article show the comparative urinary tract infection (UTI) rates in infants based on magnitude of renal dilation and antibiotic prophylaxis, respectively. The incidence of UTI was actually higher in children on prophylaxis (10% vs 8%), although infants with high-grade HN had a lower incidence on prophylaxis. Infants with reflux (23%) had a higher incidence of UTI than those without reflux (9%).

The decision to utilize prophylaxis is based on an assessment of benefits (prevent UTI, hospitalizations, renal scarring, and possibly renal insufficiency) and risks (adverse effects and bacterial resistance). As stated in the conclusion, gender, reflux and circumcision status could not be assessed in the meta-analysis. Unfortunately, these are very important factors. An infant with a normal renal ultrasound scan and high-grade reflux is at higher risk for UTI than one with high-grade hydronephrosis and no reflux. Uncircumcised boys in the first 6 months are at higher risk than those that are circumcised. Girls have a higher incidence of UTI after 6 months of age. These data can be discussed with parents to assist in developing an informed treatment plan.

D. E. Coplen, MD

High Pressure Balloon Dilation of the Ureterovesical Junction—First Line Approach to Treat Primary Obstructive Megaureter?

Garcia-Aparicio L, Rodo J, Krauel L, et al (Universitat de Barcelona, Spain)

J Urol 187:1834-1838, 2012

Purpose.—We describe the efficacy of dilation of the ureterovesical junction to treat primary obstructive megaureter.

Materials and Methods.—A total of 13 patients with primary obstructive megaureter were treated from May 2008 to December 2010. Of these patients 8 were diagnosed prenatally and the others were diagnosed after a urinary tract infection. Preoperative studies included ultrasonography, voiding cystourethrography despite vesicoureteral reflux and diuretic isotopic renogram (mercaptoacetyltriglycine). With the patient under general anesthesia, high pressure balloon dilation of the ureterovesical junction was performed under direct and fluoroscopic vision until the disappearance of the narrowed ring. A Double-J® catheter was positioned, and 2 months later it was withdrawn and the ureterovesical junction was reviewed. A secondary treatment was performed in those in whom the ureterovesical junction was still narrow. Followup was performed with ultrasonography, cystourethrography and isotopic diuretic renography.

Results.—A total of 18 procedures were performed in 13 patients (median age 7 months, range 4 to 24). Median diameter of the distal ureter was 14 mm (range 10 to 26), and median diameter of the renal pelvis and calyx was 27 mm (range 10 to 47) and 12 mm (range 9 to 26), respectively. Significant postoperative improvement of hydroureteronephrosis was observed in 11 of 13 patients and vesicoureteral reflux was found in 2. Only 3 patients needed ureteral reimplantation after endoscopic treatment due to hydroureteronephrosis in 2 and high grade vesicoureteral reflux in 1.

Conclusions.—High pressure balloon dilation of the ureterovesical junction is effective in treating primary obstructive megaureter, but long-term followup is needed.

▶ The authors report balloon dilation in infants with prenatally identified mega-ureters. Obstruction was defined by ipsilateral loss of function and not based on calculated drainage half-time (even though it was obstructive in all infants, the authors' practice pattern is observation in the presence of preserved function). There was no difficulty cannulating the narrowed segment with a 0.014 guide wire. The ureter was balloon-dilated using a 6-mm balloon for 3 minutes. A single stent was left for 2 months. A repeat dilation was performed at the time of stent removal if the pediatric cystoscope would not traverse the ureteral-vesical junction. The indication for the repeat dilation is not entirely clear because, by definition, the lumen was at least 4.8°F (surely normal in infants younger than 24 months). In infants with improved hydronephrosis, the drainage half-time normalized (< 20 minutes), and dilation resulted in reflux in a minority of infants. This approach is less invasive than open surgery but is not definitive in all infants. It requires a second anesthetic for stent removal and does not preclude subsequent surgery (open surgery is successful in 85%–90%). Balloon dilation to treat obstructed megaureters in infants and children warrants additional evaluation.

D. E. Coplen, MD

Endoscopic Management and the Role of Double Stenting for Primary Obstructive Megaureters
Christman MS, Kasturi S, Lambert SM, et al (Children's Hosp of Philadelphia, PA; Univ of Pennsylvania, Philadelphia)
J Urol 187:1018-1023, 2012

Purpose.—We determined the efficacy and potential complications of endoscopic incision and balloon dilation with double stenting for the treatment of primary obstructive megaureter in children.

Materials and Methods.—We prospectively reviewed cases of primary obstructive megaureter requiring repair due to pyelonephritis, renal calculi and/or loss of renal function. A total of 17 patients were identified as candidates for endoscopy. Infants were excluded from study. All patients underwent cystoscopy and retrograde ureteropyelography to start the procedure. In segments less than 2 cm balloon dilation was performed, and for those 2 to 3 cm laser incision was added. Two ureteral stents were placed within the ureter simultaneously and left indwelling for 8 weeks. Imaging was performed 3 months after stent removal and repeated 2 years following intervention.

Results.—Mean patient age was 7.0 years (range 3 to 12). Of the patients 12 had marked improvement of hydroureteronephrosis on renal and bladder ultrasound. The remaining 5 patients had some improvement on renal and bladder ultrasound, and underwent magnetic resonance urography revealing no evidence of obstruction. All patients were followed for at least 2 years postoperatively and were noted to be symptom-free with stable imaging during the observation period.

Conclusions.—Endoscopic management appears to be an alternative to reimplantation for primary obstructive megaureter with a narrowed segment shorter than 3 cm. Double stenting seems to be effective in maintaining patency of the neo-orifice. Followup into adolescence is needed.

▶ Most prenatally identified nonrefluxing hydroureteronephrosis resolves without loss of function or symptoms. When clinically indicated, tapered ureteral reimplantation is the gold standard for repair. Because of the very small caliber of the distal aperistaltic segment, technical issues may preclude endoscopic management in infants. The authors report on a select group of older children with a megaureter and history of urinary tract infection (UTI), urolithiasis, and diminished renal function. There is no indication whether renal scintigraphy or magnetic resonance imaging were obtained preoperatively to evaluate for obstruction. Balloon dilation alone was performed in 12 of 17 children. Postprocedure imaging showed no improvement in the dilation in the subset of 5 children having laser incision for longer narrowing. Magnetic resonance urography showed that there were no recurrent UTIs in long-term follow-up, but voiding cystourethrograms were not obtained, so it is not known if balloon dilation causes iatrogenic reflux. Endoscopic management is a less-invasive treatment option for megaureters. These preliminary results in children are encouraging.

D. E. Coplen, MD

Concomitant Endoureterotomy and Dextranomer/Hyaluronic Acid Subureteral Injection for Management of Obstructive Refluxing Megaureter

Kajbafzadeh AM, Tourchi A (Tehran Univ of Med Sciences, Iran)

J Endourol 26:318-324, 2012

Purpose.—To present the results of our experience with combined endoureterotomy and endoscopic injection of dextranomer/hyaluronic acid (Deflux) for the treatment of primary obstructive refluxing megaureter (PORM).

Patients and Methods.—Eighteen children (12 female, 6 male; mean age—14 months) with 20 PORM units underwent concomitant endoureterotomy and endoscopic subureteral Deflux injection. All patients underwent endoureterotomy at the 6-o'clock position with insertion of a 3F Double-J ureteral stent into the obstructed segment of ureter and subureteral injection of Deflux at the 5-o'clock and 7-o'clock positions. The Double-J stent was left in place with its distal tip fixed with a single knot to the external genitalia for easy removal after 1 week. Patients with refluxing nonobstructive ureter on the contralateral side of the PORM unit (seven children) underwent simultaneous endoscopic subureteral injection of Deflux. Voiding cystourethrography (VCUG) was performed at 6 months, and ultrasonography was performed at 1 week 3, 6, and 12 months postoperatively.

Results.—With a mean follow-up of 30 months, the procedure was uneventful in all patients. Follow-up VCUG showed no evidence of reflux in 15 ureterorenal (75%), significant decrease in reflux grade in 2 (10%), and no change in 3 (15%) in the endoscopic treated PORM units. No evidence of reflux was observed in the treated contralateral refluxing nonobstructive ureters. Ultrasonography revealed no ureterovesical junction obstruction. In 19 ureterorenal (95%) units, there was a complete resolution or decrease in hydroureteronephrosis.

Conclusions.—The results of this study demonstrate that combined endoureterotomy and subureteral injection of Deflux is safe and effective in the treatment of PORM in selected patients.

▶ Primary obstructive and refluxing megaureter (PORM) is a rare congenital condition with a coexisting aperistaltic segment and an ectopic-positioned (typically laterally) ureteral orifice. Although the drainage and degree of dilation typically improve in nonrefluxing megaureters, resolution of reflux is very unlikely. Tapered or imbricated ureteral reimplantation is typically performed after a year of age. The success rate (no obstruction and no reflux) after megaureter reimplantation is 90%.

The authors describe endoscopic intervention in infants with PORM and breakthrough urinary tract infection, flank pain, increasing hydronephrosis, or loss of renal function on follow-up renal scintigraphy. The endoscopic incision is at the 6 o'clock position and is down into perivesical fat. I am not sure why the incision is made through the ureteral and bladder wall. The procedure was technically not possible in one patient. The success is reasonable and approaches that of open surgery. Reflux resolved in 75%, and calculated renal scan drainage half-time was normal in all infants after surgery. The follow-up is relatively short (11–70 months). As is the case in other long-term follow-up after endoscopic injection for reflux, my suspicion is that reflux may recur in some infants.

D. E. Coplen, MD

Outcomes of fetuses with lower urinary tract obstruction treated with vesicoamniotic shunt: A single-institution experience
Ethun CG, Zamora IJ, Roth DR, et al (Baylor College of Medicine, Houston, TX)
J Pediatr Surg 48:956-962, 2013

Purpose.—The purpose of this manuscript was to examine the outcomes of patients with lower urinary tract obstruction (LUTO) treated with vesicoamniotic shunt (VAS) to improve the quality of prenatal consultation and therapy.

Methods.—The medical records of all patients diagnosed with LUTO at our center between January 2004 and March 2012 were reviewed retrospectively.

Results.—Of 14 male fetuses with LUTO, all with characteristic ultrasound findings, 11 underwent intervention. One patient received vesicocentesis alone, while 10 had VAS. Two fetuses additionally underwent cystoscopy (one with attempted valve ablation), and two had peritoneoamniotic shunts. Of 16 total VAS, 13 were placed successfully, 8 dislodged (median 7 days), and 1 obstructed (84 days). Two fetuses suffered in utero demise, and two have unknown outcomes. LUTO was confirmed in six of eight live-born fetuses. One patient died in the neonatal period, while seven survived. All six available at follow-up (median 3.7 years), had significant genitourinary morbidity. Five patients had chronic kidney disease, but only one has required dialysis and transplant. Three had respiratory insufficiency, and one required a tracheostomy.

Conclusion.—Despite significant perinatal and long-term morbidity, VAS offers patients faced with a poor prognosis an improved chance of survival. Our results underscore the need for further research into the diagnosis and treatment of LUTO.

▶ Fetal urologic intervention may be indicated in a male fetus with a normal karyotype, bladder outlet obstruction, oligohydramnios, and a normal urine sodium level ($<100 \, mEq/L$) and osmolarity ($>210 \, mOsm/L$) after serial bladder aspiration. Urinary electrolytes were not obtained in 2 fetuses and were abnormal in 2 more. Unfortunately, the authors do not correlate the postnatal renal function with the prenatal findings. Accurate prenatal diagnosis remains a concern. Lower urinary tract obstruction (urethral atresia) was confirmed in only 6 of 8 surviving infants postnatally. Although the survival rate in this series is higher than in others, the postnatal renal and pulmonary morbidity is high. Fetal intervention remains experimental and is associated with high morbidity and a need for repeat intervention.

D. E. Coplen, MD

23 Urinary Tract Infection

Urinary Tract Infection in Male Veterans: Treatment Patterns and Outcomes
Drekonja DM, Rector TS, Cutting A et al (Univ of Minnesota, Minneapolis)
JAMA Intern Med 173:62-68, 2013

Background.—Lengthier antimicrobial therapy is associated with increased costs, antimicrobial resistance, and adverse drug events. Therefore, establishing minimum effective antimicrobial treatment durations is an important public health goal. The optimal treatment duration and current treatment patterns for urinary tract infection (UTI) in men are unknown. We used Veterans Affairs administrative data to study male UTI treatment and outcomes.

Methods.—Male UTI episodes in the Veterans Affairs system (fiscal year 2009) were identified by combining *International Classification of Diseases, Ninth Revision* codes with UTI-relevant antimicrobial prescriptions. Episodes were categorized as index, early recurrence (<30 days), or late recurrence (≥30 days) cases. Drug name, treatment duration, and outcomes (recurrence and *Clostridium difficile* infection during 12 months) were recorded for index cases. Demographic, clinical, and treatment characteristics were assessed for associations with outcomes in univariate and multivariate analyses.

Results.—Among 4 854 765 outpatient male veterans, 39 149 UTI episodes involving 33 336 unique patients were identified, including 33 336 index cases (85.2%), 1772 early recurrences (4.5%), and 4041 late recurrences (10.3%). Highest-use antimicrobial agents were ciprofloxacin (62.7%) and trimethoprim- sulfamethoxazole (26.8%); 35.0% of patients received shorter-duration treatment (≤7 days), and 65.0% of patients received longer-duration treatment (>7 days). Of the index cases, 4.1% were followed by early recurrence and 9.9% by late recurrence. Longer-duration treatment was not associated with a reduction in early or late recurrence but was associated with increased late recurrence compared with shorter-duration treatment (10.8% vs 8.4%, $P < .001$), including in multivariate analysis (odds ratio, 1.20; 95% CI, 1.10-1.30). In addition, *C difficile* infection risk was significantly higher with longer-duration vs shorter-duration treatment (0.5% vs 0.3%, $P = .02$) and exhibited a similar suggestive trend in multivariate analysis (odds ratio, 1.42; 95% CI, 0.97-2.07).

Conclusion.—Longer-duration treatment (>7 days) for male UTI in the outpatient setting was associated with no reduction in early or late recurrence.

▶ This study was conducted using administrative claims data from the Veterans Affairs system and was limited to outpatients. Antimicrobial treatment was categorized as short duration (7 days or less) or long duration (more than 7 days). Most patients in the short-duration group received 7-day courses of antimicrobials, whereas most patients in the long duration group received 10-day courses. Therefore, the difference in treatment duration was not dramatically different between the groups. Nevertheless, the long-duration group exhibited a higher rate of *Clostridium difficile* infections.

This study highlights the dearth of data available to guide the management of men with urinary tract infections (UTIs). All such UTIs are considered complicated and carry a rather wide treatment recommendation of 7 to 14 days. This study suggests that a 7-day treatment course is probably adequate, but the study is far from definitive. Many potentially important factors (such as catheter use, residual urine, perioperative status) were not accounted for in the analysis.

J. Quentin Clemens, MD

Challenges in Assessing Nursing Home Residents with Advanced Dementia for Suspected Urinary Tract Infections
D'Agata E, Loeb MB, Mitchell SL (Harvard Med School, Boston, MA; McMaster Univ, Hamilton, Ontario, Canada)
J Am Geriatr Soc 61:62-66, 2013

Objectives.—To describe the presentation of suspected urinary tract infections (UTIs) in nursing home (NH) residents with advanced dementia and how they align with minimum criteria to justify antimicrobial initiation.

Design.—Twelve-month prospective study.

Setting.—Twenty-five NHs.

Participants.—Two hundred sixty-six NH residents with advanced dementia.

Measurements.—Charts were abstracted monthly for documentation of suspected UTI episodes to determine whether episodes met minimum criteria to initiate antimicrobial therapy according to consensus guidelines.

Results.—Seventy-two residents experienced 131 suspected UTI episodes. Presenting symptoms and signs for these episodes are mental status change (44.3%), fever (20.6%), hematuria (6.9%), dysuria (3.8%), costovertebral tenderness (2.3%), urinary frequency (1.5%), rigor (1.5%), urgency (0%), and suprapubic pain (0%). Only 21 (16.0%) episodes met minimal criteria to initiate antimicrobial therapy based on signs and symptoms. Of the 110 episodes that lacked minimum criteria to justify antimicrobial initiation, 82 (74.5%) were treated with antimicrobial therapy. Urinalyses and urine culture results were available for 101 episodes, of which 80 (79.2%) had positive results on both tests. The proportion of episodes with a positive urinalysis and culture was similar for those that met (83.3%) and did not meet (78.3%) minimum criteria ($P = .06$).

Conclusion.—The symptoms and signs necessary to meet minimum criteria to support antimicrobial initiation for UTIs are frequently absent in NH residents with advanced dementia. Antimicrobial therapy is prescribed for the majority of suspected UTIs that do not meet these minimum criteria. Urine specimens are frequently positive regardless of symptoms. These observations underscore the need to reconsider the diagnosis and the initiation of treatment for suspected UTIs in advanced dementia.

▶ The authors point out that, although urinary tract infections (UTIs) are common in nursing home patients, approximately one-third of cases are misdiagnosed, and, therefore, patients are overtreated. In addition, the treatment of asymptomatic bacteriuria accounts for most antimicrobial misuse in nursing homes. The challenge is differentiating whether bacteriuria is symptomatic or asymptomatic. I was pleased to discover that criteria for identifying symptomatic bacteriuria do exist—these criteria are presented in Table 1 of the original report. This study indicates that overtreatment for UTIs is particularly high in patients with advanced dementia. This is not surprising because of the limited ability to obtain a reliable history from these patients. The underlying problem is that the available test (urine culture) is sensitive but not specific for the presence of a symptomatic UTI, and the other tools we have (history, examination) are similarly nonspecific in certain populations (eg, elderly, neurogenic bladder patients). We need an additional test that can identify whether the bacteria in the urine are truly interacting with the host and causing a pathologic reaction that requires treatment, but to my knowledge no such test is forthcoming.

J. Quentin Clemens, MD

Peri-interventional antibiotic prophylaxis only vs continuous low-dose antibiotic treatment in patients with JJ stents: a prospective randomised trial analysing the effect on urinary tract infections and stent-related symptoms

Moltzahn F, Haeni K, Birkhäuser FD, et al (Univ of Bern, Switzerland)
BJU Int 111:289-295, 2013

Objective.—• To evaluate the antibiotic treatment regime in patients with indwelling JJ stents, the benefits and disadvantages of a peri-interventional antibiotic prophylaxis were compared with those of a continuous low-dose antibiotic treatment in a prospective randomised trial.

Patients and Methods.—• In all, 95 patients were randomised to either receive peri-interventional antibiotic prophylaxis during stent insertion only (group A, 44 patients) or to additionally receive a continuous low-dose antibiotic treatment until stent removal (group B, 51).

• Evaluations for urinary tract infections (UTI), stent-related symptoms (SRSs) and drug side-effects were performed before stent insertion and consecutively after 1, 2 and 4 weeks and/or at stent withdrawal.

• All patients received a peri-interventional antibiotic prophylaxis with 1.2 g amoxicillin/clavulanic acid. Amoxicillin/clavulanic acid (625 mg) once daily was administered for continuous low-dose treatment (group B).

• Primary endpoints were the overall rates of UTIs and SRSs. Secondary endpoints were the rates and severity of drug side-effects.

Results.—• Neither the overall UTI rates (group A: 9% vs group B: 10%), nor the rates of febrile UTIs (group A: 7% vs group B: 6%) were different between the groups.

• Similarly, SRS rates did not differ (group A: 98% vs group B: 96%).

• Antibiotic side-effect symptoms were to be increased in patients treated with low-dose antibiotics.

Conclusion.—• A continuous antibiotic low-dose treatment during the entire JJ stent-indwelling time does not reduce the quantity or severity of UTIs and has no effect on SRSs either compared with a peri-interventional antibiotic prophylaxis only.

▶ Should patients with an indwelling ureteral stent be on a prophylactic antibiotic? To answer this question, the authors evaluated stent placement in stone patients with a negative urine culture who were off of antibiotics at the time of placement. Most patients had stent-related symptoms (pain, hematuria, and dysuria). Unfortunately, urinary sediment and nitrite reaction were not predictive of a positive urine culture. Unless the patient is febrile or otherwise systemically ill, the decision to start antibiotics should be delayed until the urine culture results are available. Fortunately, only a small percentage of patients had a urinary tract infection (UTI) after stent placement. The foreign body does not appear to be a risk for UTI in the short time that stents are typically in place. In the absence of a history of recurrent UTIs or infectious stones, daily antibiotic use should be restricted in patients with urolithiasis requiring stent placement.

D. E. Coplen, MD

24 Pediatric Urinary Tract Infection

Different Guidelines for Imaging After First UTI in Febrile Infants: Yield, Cost, and Radiation
Scola CL, De Mutiis C, Hewitt IK, et al (Azienda Ospedaliero-Universitaria "Sant'Orsola-Malpighi," Bologna, Italy; Princess Margaret Hosp for Children, Perth, Australia; et al)
Pediatrics 131:e665-e671, 2013

Objective.—To evaluate the yield, economic, and radiation costs of 5 diagnostic algorithms compared with a protocol where all tests are performed (ultrasonography scan, cystography, and late technetium[99] dimercaptosuccinic acid scan) in children after the first febrile urinary tract infections.

Methods.—A total of 304 children, 2 to 36 months of age, who completed the diagnostic follow-up (ultrasonography, cystourethrography, and acute and late technetium[99] dimercaptosuccinic acid scans) of a randomized controlled trial (Italian Renal Infection Study 1) were eligible. The guidelines applied to this cohort in a retrospective simulation were: Melbourne Royal Children's Hospital, National Institute of Clinical Excellence (NICE), top down approach, American Academy of Pediatrics (AAP), and Italian Society of Pediatric Nephrology. Primary outcomes were the yield of abnormal tests for each diagnostic protocol; secondary outcomes were the economic and radiation costs.

Results.—Vesicoureteral reflux (VUR) was identified in 66 (22%) children and a parenchymal scarring was identified in 45 (15%). For detection of VUR (47/66) and scarring (45/45), the top down approach showed the highest sensitivity (76% and 100%, respectively) but also the highest economic and radiation costs (€52 268. 624 mSv). NICE (19/66) and AAP (18/66) had the highest specificities for VUR (90%) and the Italian Society of Pediatric Nephrology had the highest specificity (20/45) for scars (86%). NICE would have been the least costly (€26 838) and AAP would have resulted in the least radiation exposure (42 mSv).

Conclusions.—There is no ideal diagnostic protocol following a first febrile urinary tract infection. An aggressive protocol has a high sensitivity for detecting VUR and scarring but carries high financial and radiation costs with questionable benefit.

▶ The goals in infants with a history of febrile urinary tract infection (UTI) are primarily prevention of renal scarring and secondarily decreasing the morbidity of repeated urinary infections. These authors evaluated the use of 5 different diagnostic approaches in children after a first febrile UTI. Table 1 in the original article delineates the differences in the protocols. The top-down approach is the only approach that uses technetium[99] dimercaptosuccinic acid (DMSA) scintigraphy, which is much more sensitive than ultrasound in the detection of renal inflammation or abnormality. The patient population data were from the Italian Renal Infection study, which showed minimal benefit to antibiotic prophylaxis in children with low-grade reflux.

Because the top-down approach focuses on DMSA-identified renal inflammation, it is obviously most sensitive in the detection of renal scarring. Some of this scarring may not be acquired but congenital dysplasia related to high-grade reflux. Because there is some correlation between grade of reflux and renal scarring, the top-down approach misses the smallest number of patients with high-grade reflux. This analysis does not take into account that the American Academy of Pediatrics and the National Institute of Clinical Excellence algorithms recommend a voiding cystourethrogram for all children after a second febrile UTI, even in the presence of normal upper tract imaging. Although this increases the per-patient cost, it does improve the sensitivity. No perfect algorithm exists. Physicians who evaluate infants with febrile UTIs need to balance detection of all reflux with the attendant costs and the possibility of overtreating reflux when identified.

D. E. Coplen, MD

Acute ⁹⁹ᵐTc DMSA Scan Predicts Dilating Vesicoureteral Reflux in Young Children With a First Febrile Urinary Tract Infection: A Population-Based Cohort Study

Sheu J-N, Wu K-H, Chen S-M, et al (Chung Shan Med Univ Hosp, Taichung, Taiwan; China Med Univ Hosp, Taichung, Taiwan)
Clin Nucl Med 38:163-168, 2013

Objective.—This study aimed to examine the ability of acute ^{99m}Tc DMSA scan for predicting dilating (grades III-V) vesicoureteral reflux (VUR) after a first febrile urinary tract infection in children aged 2 years or younger.

Patients and Methods.—All children underwent ultrasonography (US), ^{99m}Tc DMSA scan, and voiding cystourethrography. Sensitivity, specificity, positive and negative predictive values, likelihood ratios, and receiver operating characteristic curves were performed to assess the diagnostic accuracy for predicting dilating VUR. Follow-up scan was performed at least 6 months after the acute infection to evaluate the presence of renal scarring (RS) or new scars.

Results.—Of the 473 children analyzed (289 boys and 184 girls; median age, 5 months), 282 (59.6%) had abnormal acute ^{99m}Tc DMSA scan findings. There was VUR in 153 children (32.3%), whereas 95 (20.1%) had dilating VUR. The sensitivity and negative predictive value in predicting dilating VUR were 95.8% and 97.9%, respectively, for ^{99m}Tc DMSA and 97.9% and 98.6%, respectively, for combined US and ^{99m}Tc DMSA, whereas the positive and negative likelihood ratios were 1.90 and 0.08, respectively, for ^{99m}Tc DMSA and 1.57 and 0.06, respectively, for combined studies. On multivariate analysis, dilating VUR was a predictor for developing RS and new scars.

Conclusions.—Our results reveal the usefulness of acute ^{99m}Tc DMSA scan for predicting dilating VUR in children with a first febrile urinary tract infection. A voiding cystourethrography is indicated in only children with abnormalities found on a ^{99m}Tc DMSA and/or a US. The presence of dilating VUR predisposes to developing RS and new scars.

▶ The top-down approach focuses on at-risk renal tissue as the primary indication for detection of vesicoureteral reflux. The 2011 American Academy of Pediatrics guidelines used an abnormal ultrasound scan as the primary decision point for ordering a voiding cystourethrogram. It is well known, however, that ultrasound scan is a poor predictor of reflux. A technetium dimercaptosuccinic acid (^{99m}Tc DMSA) scan is the gold standard for identification of renal inflammation. All of the infants in this study were hospitalized, and a ^{99m}Tc DMSA scan was obtained within 4 days of presentation. The presence of a positive scan in 60% of infants may be related to the severity of infection requiring hospitalization. This population may also have a higher incidence of clinically significant risk. The study confirms that high-grade reflux is a risk factor for renal inflammation and scarring. It does not address the potential morbidity of recurrent infections in the subpopulation with normal scintigraphy and lower grade reflux. Post–urinary tract infection (UTI) imaging options should be discussed with parents. The real risk of obtaining a voiding cystourethrogram in all infants with documented febrile UTI is the overtreatment of clinically insignificant abnormalities.

D. E. Coplen, MD

25 Vesicoureteral Reflux

Familial Vesicoureteral Reflux and Reflux Related Morbidity in Relatives of Index Patients with High Grade Vesicoureteral Reflux
Hunziker M, Puri P (Our Lady's Children's Hosp and Natl Children's Hosp, Dublin, Ireland)
J Urol 188:1463-1466, 2012

Purpose.—The familial nature of vesicoureteral reflux is well recognized. However, there is little information about the prevalence of vesicoureteral reflux and reflux related morbidity in the relatives of index patients with vesicoureteral reflux. Therefore, we determined the prevalence of vesicoureteral reflux and reflux related morbidity in first, second and third-degree relatives of index patients with high grade vesicoureteral reflux.

Materials and Methods.—Between 1998 and 2010 the parents of 259 index patients with grade III-V vesicoureteral reflux were asked permission to screen siblings younger than age 6 years for vesicoureteral reflux. Parents of index patients with affected siblings were contacted to obtain detailed information regarding vesicoureteral reflux, recurrent urinary tract infections, end stage renal disease, hypertension and nephrectomy among first, second and third degree relatives.

Results.—A total of 300 siblings of the 259 index patients were found to have vesicoureteral reflux on voiding cystourethrography. In terms of the other relatives of the 259 index patients 127 also had radiologically proven vesicoureteral reflux. Reflux related morbidity among the first, second and third-degree relatives included end stage renal disease in 21, nephrectomy in 12 and hypertension in 4. Of the 212 siblings who had dimercapto-succinic acid scans 49 (23.1%) showed evidence of renal scarring. In 73% of the relatives vesicoureteral reflux was seen on the mother's side.

Conclusions.—This study, the first to our knowledge, provides important information regarding reflux related morbidity in a large cohort of familial vesicoureteral reflux in first, second and third-degree relatives of index patients. Our data clearly show that there is an increased risk of reflux related morbidity among the relatives of index patients with vesicoureteral reflux and this finding has implications for counseling.

▶ Family members share common genes, with first-degree relatives (parents, children, and siblings) having 50% of genes in common and second-degree relatives (ie, aunts, uncles, nieces) sharing 25% of genes. Reflux is a multifactorial trait with an incidence that is clearly related to the degree of relationship to the index patient. The authors attempt to determine the prevalence rate in first-degree relatives of children with higher grade reflux (III—V). A voiding cystourethrography (VCUG) was obtained in all siblings less than 6 years of age, and parental assessment was typically based on history alone (ie, asymptomatic parents were not screened with a VCUG).

As anticipated, based on other studies, the incidence of reflux in siblings was more than 40%. Greater than 10% of the screened siblings had moderate-to-severe scarring on dimercaptosuccinic acid (DMSA) scan (scarring with ipsilateral renal function < 40%). There is no current evidence that screening and management of reflux will change the ultimate incidence and severity of scarring.

Sibling reflux screening is controversial. The potential downsides of a routine VCUG is detection of clinically insignificant reflux and the trauma of the actual testing. Ultrasound scan (US) is not a perfect screening tool because it is not predictive of reflux and misses small scars. However, small scars are typically clinically insignificant and not associated with hypertension and development of chronic renal insufficiency/renal failure. DMSA scintigraphy cannot be obtained in the absence of a history of urinary tract infection (UTI). The discussion of the increased risk of sibling reflux and morbidity should be discussed with parents. They can be informed that the chance of clinically significant reflux in a sibling with a normal US is small but not zero. If a VCUG is not obtained, urgent evaluation of fevers to rule out UTI is important.

D. E. Coplen, MD

Febrile Urinary Tract Infections After Ureteroneocystostomy and Subureteral Injection of Dextranomer/hyaluronic Acid for Vesicoureteral Reflux—Do Choice of Procedure and Success Matter?

Dwyer ME, Husmann DA, Rathbun SR, et al (Mayo Clinic Rochester, MN)
J Urol 189:275-282, 2013

Purpose.—Despite success rates favoring ureteroneocystostomy over subureteral injection of dextranomer/hyaluronic acid for correction of vesicoureteral reflux, the reported incidence of postoperative febrile urinary tract infection favors the latter. We evaluated contemporary treatment cohorts for an association between correction of vesicoureteral reflux and risk of postoperative febrile urinary tract infection.

Materials and Methods.—We retrospectively reviewed the records of 396 consecutive patients who underwent ureteroneocystostomy or subureteral injection of dextranomer/hyaluronic acid between 1994 and 2008. Time to event multivariate analyses included preoperative grade of vesicoureteral reflux and bladder/bowel dysfunction.

Results.—Of 316 patients meeting study criteria 210 underwent ureteroneocystostomy (356 ureters) and 106 underwent subureteral injection of dextranomer/hyaluronic acid (167). Median patient age was 5.7 years (IQR 3.4 to 8.3). Median followup was 28 months (IQR 8 to 61). Ureteral success was significantly greater after ureteroneocystostomy (88%, 314 of 356 cases) vs subureteral injection of dextranomer/hyaluronic acid (74%, 124 of 167, $p = 0.0001$). When controlling for preoperative grade of vesicoureteral reflux and bladder/bowel dysfunction, the risk of persistent reflux was 2.8 times greater after subureteral injection of dextranomer/hyaluronic acid (95% CI 1.7—4.7, $p < 0.0001$). The incidence of febrile urinary tract infection did not significantly differ between ureteroneocystostomy (8%, 16 of 210 cases) and subureteral injection of dextranomer/hyaluronic acid (4%, 4 of 106; HR 1.96, 95% CI 0.64—5.9, $p = 0.24$) even when controlling for preoperative grade of vesicoureteral reflux, a predictor of postoperative febrile urinary tract infection on multivariate analysis (HR 2.2 per increase in grade, 95% CI 1.3—3.6, $p = 0.0022$). Persistent reflux was not a predictor of postoperative febrile urinary tract infection (HR 0.81, 95% CI 0.22—2.9, $p = 0.75$ for ureteroneocystostomy vs HR 1.8, 95% CI 0.2—17.3, $p = 0.6$ for subureteral injection of dextranomer/hyaluronic acid and HR 1.8, 95% CI 0.3—3.3, $p = 0.6$ for both).

Conclusions.—The incidence of postoperative febrile urinary tract infection may be independent of radiographic procedural success.

▶ There are some studies demonstrating a decreased incidence of postoperative urinary tract infections (UTIs) after endoscopic management of vesicoureteral reflux irrespective of reflux resolution. These authors report a nonrandomized single institution evaluation of UTIs after open and endoscopic techniques. The lack of correlation of successful reflux correction and a decreased incidence of postoperative febrile UTIs drives home the point that reflux is not the only factor or mechanism that predisposes to febrile infection. Bowel and bladder dysfunctions (BBD) are associated with surgical failure. But even when a postoperative voiding cystourethrogram (VCUG) confirms reflux resolution, BBD is a huge risk factor for recurrent febrile UTIs. It is interesting that the authors state they no longer obtain postoperative VCUGs but obtain a uroflow and postvoid ultrasound in the first-line assessment of children with febrile UTIs after surgical treatment.

Onset of infections and identification of reflux after toilet training, urinary incontinence, and constipation are all factors that should drive identification and treatment of BBD prior to considering surgical intervention.

D. E. Coplen, MD

Dextranomer/Hyaluronic Acid Endoscopic Injection is Effective in the Treatment of Intermediate and High Grade Vesicoureteral Reflux in Patients with Complete Duplex Systems
Hunziker M, Mohanan N, Puri P (Our Lady's Children's Hosp and Natl Children's Hosp, Dublin, Ireland)
J Urol 189:1876-1881, 2013

Purpose.—Endoscopic subureteral injection of dextranomer/hyaluronic acid has become an established alternative to long-term antibiotic prophylaxis or surgical treatment for vesicoureteral reflux. We evaluated the effectiveness of endoscopic injection of dextranomer/hyaluronic acid in intermediate and high grade vesicoureteral reflux in patients with complete duplex collecting systems.

Materials and Methods.—A total of 123 children underwent endoscopic correction of intermediate or high grade vesicoureteral reflux using injection of dextranomer/hyaluronic acid into complete duplex systems between 2001 and 2010. Vesicoureteral reflux was diagnosed by voiding cystourethrogram, and dimercapto-succinic acid scan was performed to evaluate the presence of renal scarring. Followup ultrasound and voiding cystourethrogram were performed 3 months after the outpatient procedure and renal ultrasound thereafter every 2 years. Mean followup was 6.7 years.

Results.—Complete duplex systems were unilateral in 110 patients and bilateral in 13. Reflux severity in the 136 refluxing units was grade II in 1 (0.7%), III in 52 (38.2%), IV in 61 (44.9%) and V in 22 (16.2%). Dimercapto-succinic acid scan revealed renal functional abnormalities in 63 children (51.2%). Vesicoureteral reflux resolved after the first endoscopic injection of dextranomer/hyaluronic acid in 93 ureters (68.4%), after a second injection in 35 (25.7%) and after a third injection in 8 (5.9%). Febrile urinary tract infection developed in 5 patients (4.1%) during followup. No patient required ureteral reimplantation or experienced significant complications.

Conclusions.—Our results confirm the safety and efficacy of endoscopic injection of dextranomer/hyaluronic acid in eradicating intermediate and high grade vesicoureteral reflux in patients with complete duplex systems. We recommend this minimally invasive, 15-minute outpatient procedure as a viable option for treating intermediate and high grade vesicoureteral reflux in patients with complete duplex collecting systems.

▶ Dextranomer hyaluronic acid copolymer (Deflux) is not approved in the management of reflux in duplicated collecting systems. These authors rarely perform open ureteral reimplantation and are expanding the indications for endoscopic correction of reflux. The authors state that they excluded patients with reflux in incompletely duplicated systems but in 43 of 123 children had reflux into both moieties. In my experience, these patients have a single orifice in the bladder, and the ureters join just outside the detrusor. Management in these cases is more like those with a single ureter (and ureteral orifice). This is consistent with the authors' counting these cases as a single refluxing unit in their data analysis.

The success after a single injection (68%) in duplicated ureters is clearly lower than the authors' report after injection in singleton systems. The incidence of bowel and bladder dysfunction is amazingly low (5%) for a population of children presenting with urinary tract infections, but that may be a reason for the excellent success. The authors feel that their key to success is "injecting behind both ureteral orifices, irrespective of whether the VUR is into the lower moiety or both moieties of the complete duplex system."

Using their approach, the authors successfully reduce urinary tract infections in children with high-grade reflux and duplication. The repeated invasive testing and multiple anesthetics may not be cost-effective when compared with a single extravesical common sheath reimplantation performed on an outpatient or observation basis.

D. E. Coplen, MD

Single Center Experience with Endoscopic Subureteral Dextranomer/ Hyaluronic Acid Injection as First Line Treatment in 1,551 Children with Intermediate and High Grade Vesicoureteral Reflux
Puri P, Kutasy B, Colhoun E, et al (Natl Children's Res Centre, Dublin, Ireland; Natl Children's Hosp, Dublin, Ireland)
J Urol 188:1485-1489, 2012

Purpose. In recent years the endoscopic injection of dextranomer/ hyaluronic acid has become an established alternative to long-term antibiotic prophylaxis and the surgical management of vesicoureteral reflux. We determined the safety and effectiveness of the endoscopic injection of dextranomer/hyaluronic acid as first line treatment for high grade vesicoureteral reflux.

Materials and Methods.—Between 2001 and 2010, 1,551 children (496 male, 1,055 female, median age 1.6 years) underwent endoscopic correction of intermediate and high grade vesicoureteral reflux using dextranomer/ hyaluronic acid soon after the diagnosis of vesicoureteral reflux on initial voiding cystourethrogram. Vesicoureteral reflux was unilateral in 761 children and bilateral in 790. Renal scarring was detected in 369 (26.7%) of the 1,384 patients who underwent dimercapto-succinic acid imaging. Reflux grade in the 2,341 ureters was II in 98 (4.2%), III in 1,340 (57.3%), IV in 818 (34.9%) and V in 85 (3.6%). Followup ultrasound and voiding cystourethrogram were performed 3 months after the outpatient procedure, and renal ultrasound was performed annually thereafter. Patients were followed for 3 months to 10 years (median 5.6 years).

Results.—Vesicoureteral reflux resolved after the first, second and third endoscopic injection of dextranomer/hyaluronic acid in 2,039 (87.1%), 264 (11.3%) and 38 (1.6%) ureters, respectively. Febrile urinary tract infections developed during followup in 69 (4.6%) patients. None of the patients in the series needed reimplantation of ureters or experienced any significant complications.

Conclusions.—Our results confirm the safety and efficacy of the endoscopic injection of dextranomer/hyaluronic acid in the eradication of high grade vesicoureteral reflux. We recommend this 15-minute outpatient procedure as the first line of treatment for high grade vesicoureteral reflux.

▶ The treatment of vesicoureteral reflux is evolving. Management options include long-term antibiotic prophylaxis, surgery (endoscopic or open) correction, and observation. Endoscopic injection for correction of reflux was developed in Ireland, and this group now uses dextranomer/hyaluronic acid copolymer as a first-line treatment of grade III and IV reflux. Nearly 90% of the study population had a history of urinary tract infection. Reflux resolved after a single injection in

95% of ureters with grade III (1340) and 75% of grade IV (818). Very few of the patients had febrile urinary tract infections after injection. The authors use this as a primary therapy because parents don't like to give antibiotics and that there is no randomized trial showing efficacy. There are some short-term trials showing that most children with normal elimination patterns and reflux do well on placebo. Hopefully, the RIVUR trial will give some information regarding the utility of prophylaxis with regard to preventing infections and renal scarring. Reflux can resolve, and not all children need prophylaxis. I don't think that it is time to recommend up-front surgery in all children with reflux.

D. E. Coplen, MD

Is the Appearance of the Dextranomer/Hyaluronic Acid Mound Predictive of Reflux Resolution?
Hidas G, Soltani T, Watts B, et al (Unive of California-Irvine, Orange)
J Urol 189:1882-1885, 2013

Purpose.—After endoscopic correction of vesicoureteral reflux, we correlated the appearance of the Deflux® mound with the outcome.

Material and Methods.—We created an online survey based on 11 primary vesicoureteral reflux cases, including 6 failed and 9 successful procedures in a total of 15 renal units. Cases were selected randomly from our video library. All cases were performed by a single surgeon using the double hydrodistention implantation technique until a satisfactory mound was achieved and corrected. An online survey questionnaire was e-mailed to 234 members of the Society for Pediatric Urology. Each survey question contained a preoperative voiding cystourethrogram image as well as images of the ureteral orifice before and after injection. Respondents were asked to predict whether they thought that the appearance of the Deflux mound would be associated with successful reflux resolution on voiding cystourethrogram 3 months postoperatively. We analyzed the percent of correctly answered questions as well as the sensitivity, specificity and predictive value of the ability of experts to predict the outcome.

Results.—A total of 104 pediatric urologists responded to the survey. Overall, 66.4% of respondents predicted reflux resolution based on mound appearance, including 66% and 67% who correctly predicted success and failure, respectively. Mean outcome predictability per respondent was 66% (range 26% to 86%).

Conclusions.—The appearance of the Deflux mound and lack of hydrodistention at the completion of the procedure are not reliable predictors of outcome. Based on this experience, postoperative voiding cystourethrogram is still required to truly determine reflux resolution.

▶ The authors evaluate whether the appearance of the ureteral orifice during and immediately after Deflux injection reliably predicts resolution of vesicoureteral reflux. An online survey containing both radiographic and endoscopic images was used. In one-third of cases, success and failure were incorrectly predicted.

Although not evaluated in this study, others have found that intraoperative cystogram findings are not predictive of the absence of reflux on a cystogram 3 months after the procedure. The reasons for failure are multifactorial and include injection technique, biodegradation of the Deflux, and substrate migration. Predicting reflux resolution after endoscopic correction without a voiding cystourethrogram remains problematic.

D. E. Coplen, MD

Delayed-onset Ureteral Obstruction After Endoscopic Dextranomer/ Hyaluronic Acid Copolymer (Deflux) Injection for Treatment of Vesicoureteral Reflux in Children: A Case Series
Rubenwolf PC, Ebert A-K, Ruemmele P et al (Univ Med Centre Rogonoburg, Germany)
Urology 81:659-662, 2013

We report 4 patients with upper urinary tract (UUT) obstruction requiring ureteric reimplantation at 1, 7, 28, and 63 months after dextranomer/ hyaluronic acid copolymer (Dx/HA) injection for vesicoureteric reflux. Histopathologic evaluation of ureteric segments revealed extensive foreign body formation in all cases. We conclude that UUT obstruction is a rare but serious complication after Dx/HA injection that can occur even years after surgery. The incidence of delayed-onset UUT obstruction may be higher than previously noted. Long-term follow-up and a critical reappraisal of the method are needed to assess the late sequelae of Dx/HA injection therapy for vesicoureteric reflux.

▶ This is a concerning case series showing delayed development of ureteral obstruction after endoscopic correction of low-grade reflux. Two of the children had no dilation on the initial postoperative ultrasound scan. Subsequently, all children had marked hydroureteronephrosis, and obstruction was confirmed by MAG-3 scintigraphy, which showed no drainage. The authors injected less than 1 mL of dextranomer in all cases, but it is unlikely that the obstruction was solely related to mass effect. Presumably, the obstruction was related to progressive inflammation related to the copolymer. We don't know the denominator, but persistent reflux is clearly much more common than obstruction after endoscopic correction. Only one of the children was symptomatic. A follow-up ultrasound scan is probably indicated 12 to 24 months after dextranomer injection in asymptomatic children.

D. E. Coplen, MD

26 Cryptorchidism

Is surgical exploration necessary in bilateral anorchia?
Teo AQ, Khan AR, Williams MP, et al (Addenbrooke's Hosp, Cambridge, UK; Cambridge Univ Hosps NHS Foundation Trust, UK)
J Pediatr Urol 9:e78-e81, 2013

Objective.—To review the current management of boys with bilateral anorchia and assess whether surgical exploration is necessary when endocrine investigation indicates absent testicular function.

Patients and Methods.—The medical records of 11 boys being managed for bilateral anorchia were reviewed in relation to clinical presentation, pituitary-gonadal function, surgical and histological findings.

Results.—All boys had absence of testicular function based on undetectable levels of serum anti-Müllerian hormone, elevated basal or peak follicle-stimulating hormone and luteinising hormone levels and no testosterone response to human chorionic gonadotrophin stimulation. All boys underwent abdominal exploration, ten of whom showed no macroscopic signs of testis tissue, confirmed histologically in seven. Histology was not available in the remaining three boys. Abnormally small intra-abdominal testes were found bilaterally in one boy. These were sited in the scrotum at orchidopexy but had subsequently atrophied. Endocrine tests confirmed absent testicular function.

Conclusion.—Based on the high degree of concordance between the surgical and histological findings and the results of the endocrine tests, it is suggested that surgery is unnecessary in bilateral anorchia when endocrine tests confirm the absence of functioning testicular tissue.

▶ An infant with a normally formed phallus and bilateral nonpalpable gonads requires a neonatal evaluation to exclude Prader V virilization of a girl with congenital adrenal hyperplasia. When a 46XY karyotype is confirmed, congenital complete absence of functioning testicular tissue is very rare. Typically, the testes will at least partially descend and become palpable by 6 months of age. Ultrasound scan, computed tomography scan, and magnetic resonance imaging do not reliably conclude absence of testicular tissue. An increase in testosterone after human chorionic gonadotropin stimulation confirms the presence of functioning Leydig cells, but dysplastic testes may not respond, and the germ cells are still a malignancy risk after puberty. A markedly elevated follicle-stimulating hormone (FSH) suggests the absence of germ cells but is not 100% sensitive. The absence of anti-Müllerian hormone (AMH) indicates the absence of Sertoli cells and, by default, the absence of germ cells. The

217

authors suggest that exploration is not required when hormone tests are consistent with absence of functioning testicular tissue. Unfortunately, in this series, one patient with an undetectable AMH had small viable testes at exploration. Histology was not obtained, and the testes atrophied after orchiopexy. In this case, the baseline FSH was normal. The discordant results don't confirm absent tissue, and exploration would be indicated in this case.

D. E. Coplen, MD

Boys with Undescended Testes: Endocrine, Volumetric and Morphometric Studies on Testicular Function before and after Orchidopexy at Nine Months or Three Years of Age
Kollin C, Stukenborg JB, Nurmio M, et al (Karolinska Univ Hosp and Karolinska Institutet, Stockholm, Sweden; et al)
J Clin Endocrinol Metab 97:4588-4595, 2012

Context.—A randomized controlled study was conducted comparing the outcome of surgery for congenital cryptorchidism at 9 months or 3 yr of age.

Objective.—The aim of the study was to investigate whether surgery at 9 months is more beneficial than at 3 yr and to identify early endocrine markers of importance for testicular development.

Patients and Methods.—A total of 213 biopsies were taken at orchidopexy, and the number of germ and Sertoli cells per 100 seminiferous cord cross-sections and the surface area of seminiferous tubules and interstitial tissue were analyzed. Inhibin B, FSH, LH, and testosterone were determined. Testicular volume was assessed by ultrasonography and by a ruler.

Results.—The number of germ and Sertoli cells and testicular volume at 9 months were significantly larger than at 3 yr. The intraabdominal testes showed the largest germ cell depletion at 3 yr. At both ages, testicular volume correlated to the number of germ and Sertoli cells. None of the hormones measured during the first 6 months of life (LH, FSH, testosterone, and inhibin B) could predict the number of germ or Sertoli cells at either 9 or 36 months of age, nor could hormone levels predict whether spontaneous descent would occur or not.

Conclusion.—Morphometric and volumetric data show that orchidopexy at 9 months is more beneficial for testicular development than an operation at 3 yr of age. Testicular volume was furthermore shown to reflect germ cell numbers in early childhood, whereas endocrine parameters could not predict cellular structure ofthetestis or itsspontaneous descent.

▶ Cryptorchidism is present in 3% of full-term infants. Two-thirds of these will have testes that spontaneously descend by 6 months of age. The authors evaluate 3 groups of boys (undescended testes with spontaneous descent and those undergoing orchiopexy at 9 and 36 months of age). Histology confirms prior data showing that the number of germ cells decreases when surgery is delayed. On that basis, orchiopexy in early infancy has been recommended. Serum levels of inhibin B (Sertoli cells) and testosterone (Leydig cells) reflect production from both testes, so these have limited utility, as in most cases, the undescended testicle is unilateral. Luteinizing hormone and follicle-stimulating hormone are centrally produced, and increased levels are indicative of diminished Leydig and Sertoli cell function, respectively. There are no long-term studies showing that early surgery translates to improved fertility. However, the operation is not technically more difficult at 6 to 9 months of age, and, given the safety of anesthetics administered by pediatric anesthesiologists, there is little reason to delay orchiopexy once past the period when spontaneous descent may occur.

D. E. Coplen, MD

Growth of Spontaneously Descended and Surgically Treated Testes During Early Childhood

Kollin Č, Granholm T, Nordenskjöld A, et al (Karolinska Institutet, Stockholm, Sweden)
Pediatrics 131:e1174-e1180, 2013

Objective.—To investigate whether in congenital unilateral cryptorchidism the growth of a spontaneously descended testis is normal, compared with the contralateral scrotal testis or similar to the growth of testes that failed to descend spontaneously and later underwent orchidopexy.

Methods.—Ninety-one boys with congenital unilateral cryptorchidism with later spontaneous descent of the initially retained testis were followed from birth (0–3 weeks) up to 5 years of age and compared with boys randomized to surgery at either 9 months ($n = 78$) or 3 years ($n = 85$) of age. Testicular volume was determined with ultrasonography.

Results.—Eighty-two percent of spontaneous descent occurred before 2 months of age. Twenty-two percent of these descended testes were later again found in a retained position. The spontaneously descended testis was smaller than its scrotal counterpart at all ages ($P < .001$). We also showed a significant difference in the testicular volume between the early and late treated boys from age 2 years and onward. At 2, 4, and 5 years of age, the volumes of the spontaneously descended testes were significantly larger than those of boys operated on at 3 years but similar to those operated on at 9 months.

Conclusions.—We have shown that in boys with congenital unilateral cryptorchidism with later spontaneous descent, the originally retained testes show impaired growth compared with its scrotal counterpart from birth and onwards. Also, they are prone to later ascent to a retained position. Furthermore, the longer testes remain untreated the more they exhibit impaired growth.

▶ This study is a subset of a larger study evaluating the optimal timing of orchiopexy for undescended testes (UDT). Three percent of full-term boys have a UDT at birth. Two-thirds of testes will descend by 6 months of age. In this study, spontaneous descent occurred in a smaller percentage of infants (28%; 71 of 254) than the two-thirds reported in the literature. Most spontaneous descent occurred in the first 2 months of life. Spontaneous descent did not occur in boys randomly assigned to surgery at 3 years of age. Historically, these testes have been considered normal, but subsequent ascent (acquired UDT) occurred in 20 of 71 boys, indicating the importance of routine testicular examination during well-child visits. The volume of spontaneously descending testes was very similar to those treated with orchiopexy at 9 months of age. Early orchiopexy preserves testicular volume, and this may correlate with a more normal sperm count and fertility potential after puberty.

D. E. Coplen, MD

27 Testicular Torsion

Comparative Analysis of Detorsion Alone Versus Detorsion and Tunica
Albuginea Decompression (Fasciotomy) with Tunica Vaginalis Flap
Coverage in the Surgical Management of Prolonged Testicular Ischemia
Figueroa V, Pippi Salle JL, Braga LH, et al (Hosp for Sick Children and Univ of
Toronto, Ontario, Canada; McMaster Children's Hosp and McMaster Univ,
Hamilton, Ontario, Canada)
J Urol 188:1417-1423, 2012

Purpose.—Recent data suggest that testicular torsion may include an
element of the compartment syndrome that improves with decompression.
In 2009 we instituted tunica albuginea incision with tunica vaginalis flap
coverage as an alternative in cases in which the torsed testis continued to
appear ischemic after detorsion.

Materials and Methods.—The medical records of 65 boys who underwent scrotal exploration for testicular torsion between 2000 and 2010
were reviewed. There were 6 patients excluded from study due to lack of
followup. Of the remaining 59 patients 31 (52.5%) showed improvement
in testicular appearance after detorsion and underwent orchiopexy, whereas
28 (47.5%) did not show evidence of recovery after detorsion. Of these
patients 11 underwent tunica albuginea incision with tunica vaginalis flap
coverage and 17 underwent orchiectomy. Demographic data, duration of
symptoms and rate of testicular salvage were analyzed.

Results.—Mean patient age was 11.8 years (detorsion plus orchiopexy),
10.1 years (tunica albuginea incision plus tunica vaginalis flap coverage)
and 10.1 years (detorsion plus orchiectomy). Average followup was greater
than 6 months in all groups. Mean duration of torsion was 13.4 hours
(detorsion plus orchiopexy), 31.2 hours (tunica albuginea incision plus
tunica vaginalis flap coverage) and 67.5 hours (detorsion plus orchiectomy).
Before tunica albuginea incision with tunica vaginalis flap coverage was
offered, the rate of orchiectomy was 35.9% (14 of 39) vs 15% (3 of 20)
after this technique was introduced (p <0.05). The rates of testicular salvage
were 62.5% (detorsion plus orchiopexy), 54.6% (tunica albuginea incision
plus tunica vaginalis flap coverage) and 0% (detorsion plus orchiectomy).
Although the numbers are limited, it is likely that without tunica albuginea
incision with tunica vaginalis flap coverage 6 of 11 testes would have been
removed.

Conclusions.—This preliminary experience suggests that tunica albuginea
incision with tunica vaginalis flap coverage is a promising option for the
management of clinically marginal torsed testes, enhancing salvageability

after prolonged ischemia. We recommend considering this maneuver before performing orchiectomy in selected cases of testicular torsion.

▶ The authors describe their new surgical approach/practice pattern to improve testicular salvage in delayed presentation of testicular torsion (mean, 31 hours). Categorization of the subjective observation ("improved appearance of the testicular parenchyma after albuginea incision") that led to tunica vaginalis flap as opposed to orchiectomy cannot be ascertained. The salvage rate (< 50% testicular volume loss compared with the normal contralateral testicle) was less than 10% lower than in patients undergoing detorsion and orchiopexy alone. Intratesticular pressures were not measured before incising the tunica albuginea, so it is impossible to know if the flap had any benefit. In the presence of a normal contralateral testicle, it is unclear if this approach is better than unilateral orchiectomy.

D. E. Coplen, MD

28 Genital Ambiguity

Increased Occurrence of Disorders of Sex Development, Prematurity and Intrauterine Growth Restriction in Children with Proximal Hypospadias Associated with Undescended Testes

Sekaran P, O'Toole S, Flett M, et al (Royal Hosp for Sick Children, Glasgow, Scotland, UK)

J Urol 189:1892-1896, 2013

Purpose.—Proximal hypospadias represents 20% of hypospadias cases, which are considered to have a higher incidence of associated urological, nonurological, developmental and sexual development disorders, and chromosomal anomalies. We compared associated anomalies in boys with proximal hypospadias and undescended testis with those in boys with proximal hypospadias and descended testes.

Materials and Methods.—We reviewed the medical records of 69 boys who underwent 2-stage hypospadias repair for proximal hypospadias at a single institution during the 11-year period of 2001 to 2011. Collected data included demographics, birth history, associated urological and extra-urological anomalies, karyotype analysis and gonad palpability. Patients were divided into group 1—those with proximal hypospadias and undescended testis, and group 2—those with proximal hypospadias and descended testes. Statistical analysis was performed using the 2-tailed Fisher exact test.

Results.—There were 17 patients (25%) in group 1 with a median age of 2.2 years and 52 in group 2 (75%) with a median age of 2 years. Children in group 1 had a higher incidence of XY nondysgenetic testicular sexual development disorder (8 vs 11, $p = 0.06$), premature birth (9 vs 10, $p = 0.01$) and intrauterine growth restriction (8 each) than children in group 2 ($p = 0.01$).

Conclusions.—Prematurity and intrauterine growth restriction are significantly associated with proximal hypospadias and undescended testis. Also, due to the 28% incidence of an underlying sexual development disorder, male infants with proximal hypospadias should undergo multidisciplinary evaluation.

▶ The combination of hypospadias and undescended testes requires evaluation for a disorder of sexual differentiation (DSD). If hypospadias is present and neither testicle is palpable, this is a neonatal emergency that requires evaluation to exclude congenital adrenal hyperplasia. Less commonly, mixed gonadal dysgenesis or ovotesticular DSD are identified in boys with coexisting hypospadias and cryptorchidism. More commonly, these boys do not have an identifiable chromosomal abnormality but many have partial androgen insensitivity. In others, the coexistence is likely related to lower levels of testosterone between weeks 8 and 14 that are also associated with small gestational age and prematurity. This study clearly shows an association between intrauterine growth restriction and prematurity with under virilization in male infants.

D. E. Coplen, MD

29 Hypospadias

"Snodgraft" Technique for the Treatment of Primary Distal Hypospadias: Pushing the Envelope
Silay MS, Sırın H, Tepeler A, et al (Bezmialem Vakif Univ, Istanbul, Turkey; Sisli Etfal Training and Res Hosp, Istanbul, Turkey)
J Urol 188:938-942, 2012

Purpose.—"Snodgraft" modification has been proposed to reduce the risk of meatal/neourethral stenosis in distal hypospadias. We applied the Snodgraft technique by using inner preputial graft in primary distal hypospadias repair.

Materials and Methods.—A total of 102 consecutive patients undergoing the Snodgraft procedure were prospectively studied between 2006 and 2011. Mean patient age was 7.2 years. Localization of the meatus was glanular in 5 patients, coronal in 49, subcoronal in 45 and mid penile in 3. In all patients the posterior urethral plate was incised, and the graft harvested from the inner prepuce was sutured from the old meatus to the tip of the glans. A neourethra was created over a urethral catheter using 6-zero polyglactin suture. An interpositional flap was laid over the urethra as a second barrier. All patients were followed at 3 to 6-month intervals for cosmetic and functional results.

Results.—At a mean of 2.4 years of followup no patient had meatal stenosis or diverticulum at the inlay graft site. However, urethrocutaneous fistula was observed in 10 patients (9.8%). A slit-like appearance of neomeatus was achieved in all patients. During followup no obstructive urinary flow pattern was detected, and early and long-term maximum urine flow rates were comparable.

Conclusions.—No meatal/neourethral stenosis was observed in any patient undergoing a Snodgraft procedure. A randomized trial will be needed to prove that the incidence of meatal/neourethral stenosis is lower after Snodgraft repair compared to routine tubularized incised plate repair.

▶ Inlay grafting of the incised urethral plate is used to decrease the incidence of meatal and neourethral stenosis. Prepuce can be used for the graft in intact patients and buccal mucosa in previously operated patients. The authors utilize a preputial inlay graft in consecutive patients with very distal hypospadias (only 3 patients were proximal to the coronal margin). They give an excellent description of technique. There was no stenosis, but the fistula rate approached 10% despite the use of a dartos barrier layer. The fistulae were probably unrelated to use of the dorsal inlay graft. When tubularized incised plate urethroplasty was first introduced, there was significant concern that the incision would scar, resulting in urethral strictures. This has not been the clinical experience in large series. I don't think inlay is required in most very distal repairs. It has a definite use in reoperative repairs when the quality of the urethral plate is in question and may have a role in more proximal primary repairs.

D. E. Coplen, MD

30 Neurogenic Reconstruction

Bladder Neck Closure in Conjunction with Enterocystoplasty and Mitrofanoff Diversion for Complex Incontinence: Closing the Door for Good
Kavanagh A, Afshar K, Scott H, et al (Univ of British Columbia, Vancouver, Canada)
J Urol 188:1561-1566, 2012

Purpose.—Bladder neck closure is an irreversible procedure requiring compliance with catheterization of a cutaneous stoma and historically has been reserved for the definitive treatment of intractable incontinence after prior failed procedures. We assessed long-term outcomes of our patients undergoing bladder neck closure including continence status, additional surgical interventions, postoperative complications, conception and sexual function, and satisfaction with bladder neck closure.

Materials and Methods.—We performed a retrospective review of all patients who underwent bladder neck closure between 1990 and 2010 at our institution.

Results.—A total of 28 consecutive patients (exstrophy 15 and neurogenic bladder 13 [myelomeningocele 4, cloacal anomaly 4, spinal cord injury 2, VACTERL (Vertebral Anorectal Cardiac Tracheo-Esophageal Radial Renal Limb) 1, sacral agenesis 1 and urogenital sinus 1]) were identified. Of these patients 19 (68%) had undergone 20 unsuccessful bladder neck procedures before bladder neck closure. Bladder neck closure was initially successful in 27 of the 28 (96.4%) patients. One patient required subsequent closure of a postoperative vesicovaginal fistula. Median time from bladder neck closure was 69 months (range 16 to 250). In 11 patients 16 additional procedures were required, including stomal injection of bulking agents (2), stomal revision for stenosis (2) or prolapse (1), percutaneous nephrolithotripsy for stone (1), open cystolithotomy (2), extracorporeal shock wave lithotripsy for upper tract stones (4), repair of augment rupture (3) and open retrograde ureteral stenting for stone (1). The total surgical reintervention rate was 39.3% (11 of 28). There were no observed cases of progressive or de novo hydronephrosis.

Conclusions.—Bladder neck closure in conjunction with enterocystoplasty and Mitrofanoff diversion is an effective means of achieving continence in complex cases as a primary or secondary therapy. Long-term urological followup into adulthood is essential.

▶ Most children with neurogenic bladder secondary to congenital spinal cord anomalies have decreased bladder outlet resistance. Most can be dry with a combination of intermittent catheterization and anticholinergics. Ambulatory children often require a bladder neck procedure (fascial sling, bladder neck reconstruction, or bladder neck closure) to achieve continence. In these cases, a continent catheterizable channel is typically required because the transurethral catheterization is less reproducible after a bladder neck procedure. The potential disadvantages of bladder neck closure are an inability to access the bladder on an emergent basis if catheterization via the continent channel is not possible, the absence of a pop-off or leak point if catheterization is difficult, upper tract deterioration in the presence of complete continence and noncompliance with clean intermittent catheterization, and a theoretical higher risk of bladder perforation, although this has not been confirmed in controlled studies. The authors report short-term follow-up (median of 12 months). None of the patients had urethral leakage, but 40% required surgeries for stomal incontinence and stenosis and bladder stones that commonly develop after augmentation and reconstruction. These are not unique to bladder neck closure. There were 3 perforations, but only one was related to patient noncompliance. Bladder neck closure is a good option in patients with refractory incontinence but requires construction of a reliable catheterizable channel.

D. E. Coplen, MD

31 Neurogenic Bladder/ Urinary Diversion

Acute Spinal Cord Injury—Do Ambulatory Patients Need Urodynamic Investigations?
Bellucci CH, Wöllner J, Gregorini F, et al (Univ of Zürich, Switzerland)
J Urol 189:1369-1373, 2013

Purpose.—We compared the urodynamic parameters of ambulatory vs nonambulatory acute spinal cord injured patients.

Materials and Methods.—A total of 27 women and 33 men (mean age 58 years) with neurogenic lower urinary tract dysfunction due to acute spinal cord injury (duration of injury less than 40 days) were prospectively evaluated. The patients were dichotomized according to the mobility for moderate distances subscale of the SCIM (Spinal Cord Independence Measure) version III into ambulatory (score of 3 or greater) and nonambulatory (score less than 3). Videourodynamic parameters including maximum detrusor pressure during the storage phase, bladder compliance, detrusor overactivity, detrusor external sphincter dyssynergia and vesicoureterorenal reflux were compared between the groups.

Results.—Of the 60 patients with acute spinal cord injury 17 were ambulatory and 43 were nonambulatory. Mean ± SD duration of injury at urodynamic investigation was 30 ± 8 days. The lesion level was cervical in 14 patients, thoracic in 28 and lumbar/sacral in 18. Comparing unfavorable urodynamic parameters, no significant differences were found between ambulatory vs nonambulatory patients in terms of a high pressure system during the storage phase (29% vs 33%, $p = 0.81$), a low compliance bladder (12% vs 7%, $p = 0.54$), detrusor overactivity (24% vs 47%, $p = 0.1$), detrusor external sphincter dyssynergia (18% vs 21%, $p = 0.77$) and vesicoureterorenal reflux (0% vs 5%, $p = 0.36$).

Conclusions.—Ambulatory and nonambulatory patients with acute spinal cord injury have a similar risk of unfavorable urodynamic measures. Thus, we strongly recommend the same neurourological assessment including urodynamic investigations in all acute spinal cord injury patients independent of the ability to walk.

▶ The authors prospectively evaluate bladder function in patients with acute spinal cord injury. The patient population may represent more severe cases because the patient population was drawn from a highly specialized university injury center. Given the close proximity of somatic and autonomic systems in the spinal cord, I would expect more concordance between motor and urologic findings, but this study shows a similar incidence of elevated detrusor pressures, diminished bladder compliance, detrusor overactivity, and sphincter dyssynergia (Table 2 in the original article). Preemptive urodynamic evaluation (as opposed to observation and intervention for urinary tract infection, hydronephrosis, and other complications) may improve long-term outcomes in ambulatory SCI patients felt clinically to have a high likelihood of normal bladder function.

D. E. Coplen, MD

32 Pediatric Oncology

Lack of Specificity of Plasma Concentrations of Inhibin B and Follicle-Stimulating Hormone for Identification of Azoospermic Survivors of Childhood Cancer: A Report From the St Jude Lifetime Cohort Study
Green DM, Zhu L, Zhang N, et al (St Jude Children's Res Hosp, Memphis, TN; et al)
J Clin Oncol 31:1324-1328, 2013

Purpose.—Many male survivors of childhood cancer are at risk for azoospermia. Although both the levels of follicle-stimulating hormone (FSH) and inhibin B are correlated with sperm concentration, their ability to predict azoospermia in survivors of childhood cancer remains uncertain.

Patients and Methods.—Semen analysis was performed and serum levels of FSH and inhibin B were measured in 275 adult male survivors of childhood cancer who had received gonadotoxic therapy. Receiver operating characteristic (ROC) analysis was performed to determine the optimal inhibin B and FSH values for identifying patients with azoospermia. The patient sample was divided into a learning set and a validation set. Sensitivity, specificity, and positive and negative predictive value were calculated.

Results. Inhibin B was dichotomized as ≤ 31 ng/L or more than 31 ng/L and FSH was dichotomized as ≤ 11.5 mIU/mL or more than 11.5 mIU/mL based on results of the ROC analysis. Using these values, the specificity of the serum level of inhibin B for identifying azoospermic survivors was 45.0%, and the positive predictive value was 52.1%. The specificity for FSH was 74.1%, and the positive predictive value was 65.1%.

Conclusion.—Neither serum inhibin B nor FSH is a suitable surrogate for determination of sperm concentration in a semen sample. Young men and their physicians should be aware of the limitations of these measures for assessment of fertility potential.

▶ Long-term effects become important as the treatment of childhood and adolescent cancer improves. Both irradiation and chemotherapeutic alkylating agents will alter spermatogenesis. Semen analysis can estimate fertility potential, but producing a sample may be problematic for age-related and social or religious reasons. The level of inhibin-B is inversely related to follicle stimulating hormone, which is inversely related to sperm concentration in healthy males. These authors evaluated these parameters in adult male cancer survivors (median age 30.5 years, range 19 to 57 years). The poor specificity and positive predictive value limit the use in differentiating azoospermia from normal counts. Sexually active males need to understand that, regardless of the level of the biomarkers, protection should be used during intercourse if pregnancy is not desired.

D. E. Coplen, MD

33 Pediatric Laparoscopy/ Reconstruction

Laparoscopic Pyeloplasty for Ureteropelvic Junction Obstruction in Infants
Turner RM II, Fox JA, Tomaszewski JJ, et al (Children's Hosp of Pittsburgh of Univ of Pittsburgh Med Ctr, PA)
J Urol 189:1503-1507, 2013

Purpose.—Laparoscopic pyeloplasty and open pyeloplasty have comparable efficacy for ureteropelvic junction obstruction in pediatric patients. The role of laparoscopic pyeloplasty in infants is less well defined. We present our updated experience with laparoscopic pyeloplasty in children younger than 1 year.

Materials and Methods.—We retrospectively reviewed the records of all 29 infants treated with transperitoneal laparoscopic pyeloplasty for symptomatic and/or radiographic ureteropelvic junction obstruction from May 2005 to February 2012. Patients were followed with renal ultrasound at regular intervals. Treatment failure was defined as the inability to complete the intended procedure, persistent radiographic evidence of obstruction and/ or the need for definitive adjunctive procedures.

Results.—Transperitoneal laparoscopic pyeloplasty was performed in 29 infants 2 to 11 months old (mean age 6.0 months) weighing 4.1 to 10.9 kg (mean ± SD 7.9 ± 1.6). Followup was available in all except 5 patients (median 13.9 months, IQR 7.7–23.8). Mean operative time was 245 ± 44 minutes. All cases were completed laparoscopically. Three postoperative complications were reported, including ileus, superficial wound infection and pyelonephritis. Two patients had persistent symptomatic and/or radiographic evidence of obstruction, and required reoperative pyeloplasty. The overall success rate was 92%.

Conclusions.—Laparoscopic pyeloplasty in infants remains a technically challenging procedure limited to select centers. Our early experience revealed a success rate comparable to that of other treatment modalities with minimal morbidity.

▶ The authors were early adopters of laparoscopic dismembered pyeloplasty in infants and children with ureteropelvic junction obstruction. The authors report on a subset of patients less than one year of age (of 139 children in a 7-year period). The success is good, but the laparoscopic magnification did not result in improved outcomes when compared with series of open pyeloplasty. The series is small, and with only 2 failures it is difficult to ascertain technical factors that contributed to persistent obstruction. Laparoscopic pyeloplasty in infants is safe and feasible. The advantages of this approach in infants are not clearly defined.

D. E. Coplen, MD

Cost Analysis of Pediatric Robot-Assisted and Laparoscopic Pyeloplasty
Casella DP, Fox JA, Schneck FX, et al (Children's Hosp of Pittsburgh, PA)
J Urol 189:1083-1086, 2013

Purpose.—An increasing percentage of pediatric pyeloplasties are being performed with assistance of the da Vinci® Surgical System. A review of the recent literature shows decreased operative times and length of hospital stays when robotic procedures are performed, although there are few published data comparing the cost of pediatric robotic and pure laparoscopic pyeloplasty. We reviewed a representative sample of pyeloplasties performed at our institution and performed a cost analysis.

Materials and Methods.—We retrospectively identified 23 robot-assisted and 23 laparoscopic pyeloplasties performed at our institution between August 2008 and April 2012. Total cost was calculated from direct and indirect costs provided by our billing department.

Results.—Robotic procedures were shorter than pure laparoscopic procedures (200 vs 265 minutes, $p < 0.001$) but there was no significant difference in the total cost of the 2 procedures ($15,337 vs $16,067, $p < 0.46$). When compared to laparoscopic cases, subgroup analysis demonstrated decreased operative times (140 vs 265 minutes, $p < 0.00001$) and total cost ($11,949 vs $16,067, $p < 0.0001$) in robotic cases where stents were placed in an antegrade fashion.

Conclusions.—With widespread use the cost of robotic instrumentation may decrease, and experience may further shorten operative times. However, it currently remains to be seen whether robotic technology will become a cost-effective replacement for pure laparoscopy in the management of pediatric ureteropelvic junction obstruction.

▶ The authors compare the costs between laparoscopic and robotic-assisted pediatric pyeloplasty. As expected, there was no difference in the postoperative hospitalization and convalescence. They do not report or factor clinical outcomes into the data, but failures requiring reoperation would clearly increase costs. Operating times were shorter with robotic assistance, but the added cost of the robotic supplies gave comparable expenses. At this institution, the expense of acquiring and maintaining the robot is equally charged against all surgical cases. If those costs were unilaterally applied to robotic cases, then robotic case volumes would need to increase significantly to maintain comparable costs. Unless hospital length of stay is shorter after more complex robotic reconstructions, there will not be a cost advantage achieved with robotic assistance. Equivalent costs and clinical outcomes are okay, but hospital systems will need to continue to grapple with the trade-off between the cost of new technologies when compared with existing treatment approaches with excellent clinical outcomes.

D. E. Coplen, MD

Endopyelotomy for Pediatric Ureteropelvic Junction Obstruction: A Review of our 25-Year Experience
Kim EH, Tanagho YS, Traxel EJ, et al (Univ School of Medicine, St Louis, MO)
J Urol 188:1628-1633, 2012

Purpose.—We elucidate the role of endopyelotomy as a primary and secondary intervention for ureteropelvic junction obstruction in children.

Materials and Methods.—We retrospectively identified 79 pediatric patients who underwent endopyelotomy for ureteropelvic junction obstruction between 1986 and 2011. Eleven patients were lost to followup and were excluded from analysis. Patient demographics, operative information, complications and success rates were reviewed for the remaining 68 patients. Treatment success was defined as the absence of symptom recurrence and improved radiographic features on ultrasound, computerized tomography, diuretic renogram or excretory urogram at most recent followup.

Results.—Primary endopyelotomy data were analyzed in 37 patients with a median age of 11.1 years. The success rate was 65% at a median followup of 34 months (range 1.5 to 242). Treatment failure occurred in 13 patients with a median time to failure of 8 months (range 1.5 to 131). There were 8 cases of failure during 12 months of surgery. Secondary endopyelotomy data were analyzed in 31 patients with a median age of 6.5 years. The success rate was 94% at a median followup of 61 months (range 1 to 204). Treatment failure occurred in 2 patients at 1 and 6 months. Approximately two-thirds of all procedures used an antegrade approach.

Conclusions.—Primary endopyelotomy is significantly less successful than pyeloplasty in the treatment of ureteropelvic junction obstruction in pediatric patients. However, secondary endopyelotomy following failed pyeloplasty represents a viable alternative to redo pyeloplasty.

▶ Endopyelotomy for management of ureteropelvic junction obstruction was first described in the 1980s by Mr J.E.A. Wickham. In adult patients primary success was 60% to 70%, and this minimally invasive approach had been supplanted by laparoscopic dismembered pyeloplasty. Open dismembered pyeloplasty remains the gold standard in children, although laparoscopic repair clearly has less morbidity in older children. Because of issues with ureteral and instrument size, there are very few series of endopyelotomy in children. The authors show poor results when endopyelotomy is used as a primary modality in pediatric ureteropelvic junction obstruction. However, the outcomes are markedly improved when endopyelotomy is used in recurrent/persistent obstruction after prior pyeloplasty.

The improved outcomes are likely related to management/elimination of a crossing vessel at the time of pyeloplasty; creation of a funneled, dependent ureteropelvic junction; and perhaps reduction of the renal pelvis. Retrograde access may be difficult in an infant, but prestenting will usually eliminate this concern. If a nephrostomy tube has already been placed, then antegrade incision is technically easy. This approach is less invasive than either an open or laparoscopic dismembered pyeloplasty.

D. E. Coplen, MD

Article Index

Chapter 1: Clinical Outcomes

Chapter 2: Imaging

Chapter 3: Quality Improvement

Chapter 4: Clinical Research

Chapter 5: Endourology and Stone Disease

Chapter 6: Transplantation

Chapter 7: Trauma

Chapter 8: Female Urology

Chapter 9: Benign Prostatic Hyperplasia

Chapter 10: Male Incontinence/Voiding Dysfunction

Chapter 11: Voiding Dysfunction/Enuresis

Chapter 12: Sexual Function

Chapter 13: Hypogonadism

Chapter 14: STD

Chapter 15: Renal Tumors

Chapter 16: Prostate Cancer

Chapter 17: Bladder Cancer

Chapter 18: Urinary Reconstruction

Chapter 19: Infertility

Chapter 20: Varicocele

Chapter 21: Pediatric Urology

Chapter 26: Cryptorchidism

Chapter 27: Testicular Torsion

Chapter 28: Genital Ambiguity

Chapter 29: Hypospadias

Chapter 30: Neurogenic Reconstruction

Chapter 31: Neurogenic Bladder/Urinary Diversion

Chapter 32: Pediatric Oncology

Chapter 33: Pediatric Laparoscopy/Reconstruction

Author Index

Printed and bound by CPI Group (UK) Ltd, Croydon, CR0 4YY

08/05/2025

01864755-0003